Why Dementia Makes Communication Difficult

Why Dementia Makes Communication Difficult

A Guide to Better Outcomes

ALISON WRAY

Jessica Kingsley Publishers
London and Philadelphia

First published in Great Britain in 2021 by Jessica Kingsley Publishers
An Hachette Company

1

Copyright © Alison Wray 2021
Illustrations copyright © David Hallangen 2021

The right of Alison Wray to be identified as the Author of the Work has been
asserted by her in accordance with the Copyright, Designs and Patents Act 1988.

A CIP catalogue record for this title is available from the
British Library and the Library of Congress

ISBN 978 1 78775 606 9
eISBN 978 1 78775 607 6

Printed and bound by CPI Group (UK) Ltd, Croydon, CR0 4YY

Jessica Kingsley Publishers' policy is to use papers that are natural,
renewable and recyclable products and made from wood grown in
sustainable forests. The logging and manufacturing processes are expected
to conform to the environmental regulations of the country of origin.

Jessica Kingsley Publishers
Carmelite House
50 Victoria Embankment
London EC4Y 0DZ

www.jkp.com

Contents

Acknowledgements

This book distils and (I hope) makes more accessible the main content of my lengthy academic text *The Dynamics of Dementia Communication* (Oxford University Press, 2020). The many people who contributed to the development of those ideas are acknowledged there, but those whose examples or ideas feature here deserve mention: Samantha Collins, David Green, Wendy Lewis, Danuta Lipinska, Rois McDonagh, Lydia Morris and Val Ormrod. The book has benefited from the generosity of five people who carefully read and fed back on the draft: Phil McEvoy, Maria Nicol, Val Ormrod, Alister Robertson and Pauline Strong. Between them, these individuals represent my main target reader groups – dementia care professionals, carer trainers, allied health professionals, family members and people who are themselves living with a dementia. To all of you, thank you for your insightful observations and your support for this enterprise. I'm grateful to illustrator David Hallangen for generously allowing me to use images from our animated films.[1] I'd also like to thank my husband, Mike Wallace, who heard many of the ideas first (and probably came up with a few of them). Finally, thank you to Adam Renvoize for his work on the cover design, and to Elen Griffiths, Emma Scriver and Claire Robinson at Jessica Kingsley Publishers for guiding me through the practicalities of writing this sort of book.

---

1   Wray (2017, 2018, 2020a)

Preface: What Is This Book About and Is It for You?

Dementia brings many challenges. None, however, is greater than its effect on communication. Dementia can cause difficulties with finding words, following conversations and recalling what's been said and what's happened. It can also affect a person's ability to piece together the different bits of information needed for creating and understanding statements and questions. Because communication is so important for our daily activities and our relationships, any problems with it can quickly impact negatively on our quality of life. And because communication is something we do with others, if dementia creates challenges for one person in the conversation, everyone's affected.

If you've experienced, or are simply interested in, how dementia changes communication, then this book has been written for you. Perhaps you have a dementia diagnosis yourself and are concerned about being able to communicate effectively in the future. Perhaps you have a family member living with a dementia and want to support them better, as well as learn to manage your own responses to the things they say and the challenges they face. Perhaps your job involves supporting people living with a dementia every day. Or perhaps you just encounter them occasionally through your work as, say, a hairdresser, shop assistant, religious leader, taxi driver, plumber or postal delivery worker. If so, you might be wondering how best to complete your tasks while helping them feel comfortable around you. Perhaps you have a neighbour or friend with a dementia diagnosis, and wish you knew what to say to them, and how to be more supportive without experiencing any awkwardness and embarrassment. Or you might simply be interested in how communication works and why dementia makes it go wrong.

No book can solve all the problems, because every person is different and every dementia is different. So, although there are plenty of suggestions and ideas in these pages, the main purpose of the book is to explain *why* communication is so badly damaged by dementia. The best person to fix your communication problems is you, at the time they happen. For that, you need to recognize what's going on, and know what the options are for how to respond. There's no magic wand, unfortunately. But this book can help you develop insights and ideas to try out.

CHAPTER ONE

Introduction

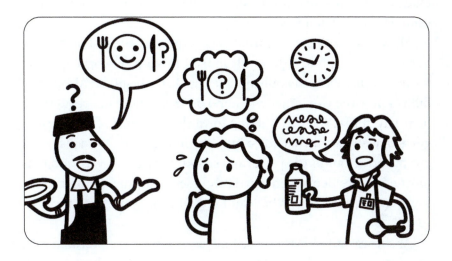

Kenny

I was waiting in the lobby of a residential care home while a staff member hunted for information about the facilities. It was a Sunday afternoon, and my husband was with me because this wasn't a work visit. We were on a reconnaissance mission – my mother, at very short notice, had turned the corner from living independently to needing residential care, and we were wondering if this was the right place for her.

The building was old, with high ceilings, cornices and an air of grandeur. The lobby was in the former grand entrance hall, at one end of which a reception desk had been set up. The only staff member in the room was hidden behind the desk, bending down to search through a cupboard. Around me, several residents were sitting in high-backed armchairs, snoozing or watching the world go by. Sounds typical of residential care homes echoed around the lobby, despite the furnishings, carpet and full-length curtains – shuffles of movement, squeaks of equipment, conversation, the occasional distressed shout or scream and, from the adjacent dining room, the clinking of cups as afternoon tea and cake were served.

From my left, I heard a voice, and caught a movement in my peripheral vision. An elderly lady had stood up from her chair and taken a few steps forward using her wheeled Zimmer frame, while calling to me, 'Help me, help me.'

I looked over at the reception desk, expecting the staff member's head to pop up, but it didn't. It looked for all the world as if my husband and I were the only non-residents in the place. Although I didn't know the woman, it was impossible to ignore her request for help. Given that she was walking towards me, I made the educated guess that she would like to go into the dining room. We'd just been given a brief tour of the place, and so I knew where it was, and that most of the residents were currently assembled there. I took a step towards her, and said, 'What can I do? Did you want to go through to tea?'

As she was still slowly proceeding towards me, I reciprocated with a few more steps in her direction, and when I reached her, she took my hand, and said, 'Whatever you want, take it. I just wanted to say.'

Since she hadn't answered my question, but rather appeared to be offering me advice, I wasn't sure how to reply. So, I just said, 'Yes?'

'That's what I want you to do,' she said. 'Whatever you want, you should take it. Have it. That's what...' Her sentence concluded with a few words I couldn't catch.

'Well,' I replied, 'thank you. That's good to know.'

I knew it was a bit lame, but I wasn't sure what else to say. It didn't occur to me to ask her what sort of thing she thought I should take or have, or why it was important. I was too focused on myself and my own awkwardness. But I did want to continue with the conversation, so I decided to change the subject to something I'd have a little more control over.

'What's your name?' I asked her.

'Well...' she said, and then went quiet for several seconds.

Oh dear, I thought, *now I've put her on the spot. Perhaps she can't recall her name any more.* How wrong I was. What she seems to have been doing was deciding which name to tell me, because when she finally replied, she said, 'They call me Kenny.' (Actually, she didn't say *Kenny*. For reasons of privacy, I've changed the name, as I have with all such examples in this book. But it was a name with similar characteristics.)

In other words, she gave me her nickname. She'd chosen to engage at this informal level with me, rather than telling me her given name or title and surname. *Kenny* isn't the sort of name you expect an elderly lady in Britain to have, because it sounds like a diminutive of *Kenneth*, a man's name. So, I said, 'Kenny? That's an unusual name.'

'My brother gave me that name,' she replied.

Now, here was an opportunity for an interesting conversation. I could have asked how that came about or got her to tell me more about her brother. Perhaps we'd have ended up talking about her childhood, which was probably during the Second World War. I could have asked her if she had a nickname for him as well. It's possible that she'd have struggled to sustain such a conversation, but I'll never know, because I didn't even think to try. Instead, I closed the topic down with, 'That's nice.' And then I steered the conversation back to my agenda. I was on a mission. I was going to solve her problem (as I saw it).

'Now, Kenny,' I said, 'shall I help you go and get your tea? You seem to be on your way somewhere.'

'No,' she said. 'Just to see you. I wanted to see you and tell you.'

'Well,' I replied, 'thank you, Kenny. That was really kind of you.' And with that, she slowly turned herself around and walked back to her seat.

As soon as I could, I grabbed paper and a pen and wrote the conversation down, because I could see it had a lot to teach me. I'd not managed things at all well. By making hasty, unnecessary assumptions, I'd fallen into a set of traps I might have avoided. I was so focused on my own awkwardness about not being sure what Kenny meant, that I'd ended up totally misunderstanding what was going on. She didn't want to go to the dining room for tea. As my husband pointed out afterwards (for I had completely failed to notice), there was a small table next to her chair, on which a cup of tea and a piece of cake were already sitting.

What motivated Kenny to call out to me and make the effort of standing up and coming towards me? We'll never know. Nor can we know exactly what her advice was supposed to be. But what's clear is that she went to a lot of effort to achieve something of importance to her. Perhaps her aim was to give me advice she wished she'd followed herself in the past. Or she might have wanted to do something for a stranger, to be useful, to make a difference – a rather similar goal to my own, then. Perhaps she thought I looked lost and she wanted to reassure me. Maybe she just wanted to strike up a conversation, in an environment where it was certainly possible to feel alone despite having others around her.

In all events, she had an agenda, which she stuck doggedly to, though she got little help or appreciation from me. I had an agenda as well. Indeed, I had more than one: to help this poor old lady to get tea she didn't need; to be nice to her (although doing that by ignoring what she said perhaps wasn't the best method); to minimize my own embarrassment; and to control the conversation, because that made *me* feel better.

Probably, neither of us actually achieved quite as much as we wanted, because we tripped over each other, metaphorically speaking. I was clumsy, while she, because of her dementia, was unable to provide enough information to make her statement meaningful for me. Both of us were trying to make changes to our immediate situation, our experiential world. But neither of us could do so without getting the other to do something on our behalf, and in this, we both had only limited success.

Yet on the surface, it looked like an engaged conversation. We took turns. Questions and statements were exchanged and were answered and acknowledged. Someone passing by might have thought, *How lovely to see Kenny having a nice chat.* I don't know how *she* felt at the end of it, but I, certainly, emerged feeling dissatisfied, awkward and a little guilty.

What could I have done differently? It's perhaps not so much a question of the details, such as exactly what I did or didn't say, but of my overall approach. I needed to be more alert to what Kenny was trying to achieve. And I needed greater awareness of how my own priorities were shaping what I did and didn't say. Only with such awareness would I have been able to see where I had opportunities for choice and to weigh up the pros and cons of each option.

Probably, I'd never have entirely escaped my own agendas, but I could have noticed and questioned them, and broadened the range of things that I'd be happy to achieve in this interaction. I needed to be more sensitive to the clash between what Kenny said and what I expected her to say, and how that clash shaped what happened next. This sort of insight isn't easy to come up with in real time. But by studying how communication works – what drives it, and what determines how we choose to express ourselves – we can develop a deeper instinct for what might be going on and what might work.

Let's consider a couple of examples from my conversation with Kenny. I was put on the back foot by the first thing she said. Why did she ask for help when she only wanted to tell me something? We can't know, but it may have been something she'd learned within her residential home environment: if you just say *Excuse me*, you get ignored. Asking for help is a more effective way to get attention. If so, then her choice was appropriate and sensible in her context. It indicates that, despite her dementia, she was capable of taking stock of a situation and adapting to it.

And then, when I asked if she wanted to go through to the dining room for tea, why didn't she tell me she had tea and cake already, or point to the table with the cup and plate? That's how we usually play the interaction game – we spot when the other person has made a false assumption and we correct it. Then we both know where we are. If she'd done that, I'd have given up on that assumption and focused more quickly on her actual statement.

But Kenny was living with a dementia. Perhaps she couldn't recall that she'd got tea and cake. Perhaps she couldn't put herself in my shoes, to realize what I was assuming. When there's a conversation between a person who's living with a dementia and someone who isn't, it's not a level playing field. That's not to say that people living with a dementia can't also help themselves in various ways, as we'll see. But the person without a dementia should be ready to pick up more of the strain when the communication doesn't work optimally. That's the lesson I learned from my encounter with Kenny, and it's one of the key messages of this book.

Pinning down communication and dementia

The quality and effectiveness of communication play a major role in how well people living with a dementia manage. The same applies to their family and friends, to care professionals and anyone else who interacts with them. None of us like it when communication doesn't work very well. So, one of the things this book aims to do is explain how communication operates. That will make clearer just how it can be disrupted and what effects the disruption has. With that information it'll be easier to think about how changes in our approach to communication can make a positive difference.

Communication lies at the heart of almost everything we do. It's obviously central when we're chatting to someone or using social media, but there's so much more to it than that. Road signs are a form of communication. So are the electronic boards that announce the next train, bus or tram, and the 'open' and 'closed' signs on the doors of shops. When we read a book, the author is communicating with us. We also observe and, in a sense, participate in, the communication between characters or presenters in films, TV and radio programmes.

As for the everyday objects we use, the designers, manufacturers, instruction writers and advertisers all communicate with us. Furthermore, we talk to our pets and may try to interpret the behaviour of wild animals in terms of communication. Even when we're thinking, we're communicating with ourselves. As a result, if the mechanisms of communication are upset, everything's upset. And given the many ways that dementia can interfere with communication, it's no wonder that people living with a dementia can so easily feel disorientated and anxious.

It makes sense, then, that when we look for ways to improve the experience of those living with a dementia and the many people who interact with them, we should examine how communication is working, and whether it could work better. This isn't the first book to address communication, but it goes a lot deeper than many. Rather than only offering tips on what to say and how to say it, this book explores the underlying motivations of communication, so we can better understand why we say what we do, why we say it the *way* we do, what can go wrong and how attempts to fix things can go awry. It looks at the choices we make and where there's most scope for making different choices.

The book is relevant not only to family members and professionals in support roles, but also to people living with a dementia themselves. One of the things that's struck me over the time I've been working in this field is how little guidance there is for people living with a dementia, about how to help *themselves*. People given a cancer diagnosis are talked through what will happen next and advised on their options and priorities. People diagnosed with heart disease or type 2 diabetes are given guidance on changes they need to make to their daily lifestyle, so as to live better with their illness. When someone has a stroke, they get advice on what to do to maximize their chances of a good recovery. But when people get a dementia diagnosis, there's far less on offer. If anyone's given advice at all, it's often the person they're with – their spouse, son or daughter. Yet, particularly as scientific advances make it possible to diagnose dementia earlier, a great many of those who receive a dementia diagnosis are perfectly capable of taking on some responsibility for making plans and adjustments. There's plenty that they can do that could have long-term benefits for their experience of communication in the future. With that in mind, at the end of each chapter there are practical tips not only for family, friends and professional carers, and for more casual bystanders, but also for people living with a dementia themselves.

I hope that this book will contribute to answering some of the questions that are commonly asked about dementia, such as:

QUESTIONS ABOUT DEMENTIA

Questions people living with a dementia diagnosis might ask:

– What steps can I take now that will help me later?
– How can I avoid getting isolated and depressed?
– What should I be asking my family and friends to do to support me?
– Why do my memory lapses make me feel so vulnerable?
– Am I still going to be the same person I am now?
– Should I mind if people don't always tell me the truth?

Questions professionals, family members and friends might ask:

– Is this the same person I used to know?
– What's the best way to help the person feel secure, confident and calm?
– Why does the person's forgetfulness annoy me so much?
– What should I do if I don't know what s/he's saying or if s/he can't understand me?
– What can I do if I find communication embarrassing and awkward?
– Why do I feel so guilty even though I'm doing my best?
– How much should I expect of her/him?
– Is it okay to lie to her/him?

Outline of the book

In the rest of this chapter, we explore what 'dementia' is and what causes it, before looking at how it affects the cornerstone of communication – language.

Chapter 2 looks at four types of *reserve*. These reserves are biological, behavioural, environmental and personal resources. They determine how much protection people have against dementia and its symptoms. We'll explore how decisions we make can increase our own and others' level of reserve.

Chapter 3 gets to the heart of how communication actually works. Why do we communicate? What is involved in communicating?

This helps us see where the potential weak points are – the places where dementia can get a hold, both the obvious ones and the less obvious ones.

Chapter 4 digs more deeply into what it takes to communicate effectively and explores the role of memory in communication. Not all types of dementia feature difficulties with memory, but, one way or another, most of them do. We'll see that there is a lot more to it than just difficulties recalling someone's name or forgetting what you were about to say.

In Chapter 5, we home in what happens when communication goes wrong due to dementia. It'll become clear that difficulties with words, grammar and pronunciation are not the major problem. Rather, communication breaks down when the speaker and listener aren't sure what the other person knows already.

Chapter 6 explores those awkward moments when we don't know what to say in reply, because we're not sure what the other person meant. We'll see that these situations can easily undermine everyone's confidence, so it's important to have tactics for dealing with them.

Chapter 7 asks whether dementia changes someone into a different person. With a focus still on communication, it shows why it's so challenging to find our way between expecting everything to be as it was and assuming that the person is less able than they actually are.

Chapter 8 tackles an issue of major concern to many people living with a dementia and those who love and care for them – whether it's acceptable to lie, if we believe doing so is in the person's interests. It's a question that divides people, but we'll look beneath the surface, at the various reasons why deception can be seen as a good and a bad thing. This offers some pointers for how to make appropriate choices.

Chapter 9 draws together the previous ideas to focus on a range of ways in which we can all help make communication work better.

A note or two on the terminology used in the book might be helpful here. In recognition of their preferences, I use the term *people living with a dementia* rather than *people with dementia*. This helps us remember that no one should be defined purely according to that one characteristic. Dementia is something people deal with as they live their lives, rather than the sum of who they are. Next, what's the most appropriate way to describe the various people who support people living with a dementia? Terms in common use include: *carer, caregiver, supporter, support person, enabler* and *care partner*. In this book I've chosen to use *carer* to refer to those providing physical and social support, whether they're professionals or family members. However, I often use *carers and families*, which helps signal that family members have other roles too. The aim is to remain clear about who I mean, and to keep the focus firmly on communication, which transcends roles and relationships, even if it's often shaped by them. Main terms related to dementia are explored in the next section and other concepts are defined as they arise.

What is dementia?

Dementia isn't just one thing. There are several types, with different causes and characteristics. Furthermore, two people with the same diagnosis might not have all the same symptoms or might have symptoms to different extents. We'll come back later to why that is. But before that, it'll be useful to get some markers down about what's what.

First, we need to separate out some terms and concepts that easily get very confusing. For a start, what does *dementia* mean and how does it relate to terms like *Alzheimer's disease*? *Dementia* is a troublesome word. To get to the root of the problem we have to distinguish between *illnesses*, which are caused by, say, an injury, genetically based changes or bacteria, and *symptoms*, which are caused by the illnesses.

Technically, the word *dementia* refers to the symptoms of illnesses like Alzheimer's disease. But, rather unhelpfully, some of the illnesses that can cause dementia have the word *dementia* in their name, including 'vascular dementia', 'fronto-temporal dementia' and 'dementia with Lewy bodies'. In one sense it doesn't matter, because the illnesses are typically only diagnosed via the symptoms. In other words, by the time someone has an illness with *dementia* in its name, they have some symptoms that can be termed 'dementia' as well. But it's important to note that having one of the underlying illnesses doesn't in itself predict the severity and progression of dementia *symptoms*, as we'll see in Chapter 2.

Regarding the different dementia-causing diseases, the four main ones are: Alzheimer's disease, vascular dementia, Lewy body spectrum disorder and fronto-temporal dementia (however, the latter two have several different forms and names, which can be confusing). The underlying causes of these four diseases are imperfectly understood, but we do know that vascular dementia is associated with strokes or mini-strokes (transient ischaemic attacks, or TIAs). Motor neurone disease can cause a form of fronto-temporal dementia, and Parkinson's disease can lead to a form of Lewy body spectrum disorder.

Alzheimer's disease is the most commonly diagnosed dementia-causing disease, and, according to the World Health Organization[1] affects 60–70 per cent of those living with a dementia. Its cause is still under investigation, but the damage in the brain includes 'plaques' of amyloid and 'tangles' of tau – two types of abnormality that prevent the brain cells communicating with each other. Furthermore, the brain as a whole also starts to shrink. The damage caused by Alzheimer's appears to begin in the hippocampus, which is the brain area responsible for turning our temporary memory of something that's just happened into a more permanent record. That's why one of the first noticeable symptoms of Alzheimer's is not being able to recall some event from earlier in the day.

Neither Alzheimer's nor any other type of dementia will look the same in everyone. Labels are stuck onto various parts of a very complicated set of characteristics to help doctors and researchers make some sort of sense of them. But, increasingly, specialists believe that rather than thinking of the dementia-causing diseases as clear landmarks, we should see them as part of a landscape that gradually changes from, say, flat to hilly, or from sandy to rocky, without there being a precise place where one type of terrain finishes and another starts. In other words, it may not always be possible to say that

---

1   www.who.int/news-room/fact-sheets/detail/dementia

someone has a particular type of dementia, or even a specific disease that's causing it, because that person might have characteristics that cut across the way we currently label the conditions.

We're all different. It's not surprising, then, that even if the dementia-causing diseases really were distinct from each other, which they seem not to be, then the manifestations of those diseases would vary from person to person. As we'll see in Chapter 2, one reason seems to be that we vary in how well we can withstand either the dementia-causing diseases themselves or the symptoms they can cause.

How does dementia affect language?

We've just seen that the different types of dementia are difficult to fully separate if we focus on symptoms. This is very evident when it comes to communication. While each variety of dementia is generally associated with different types of difficulty, not all of the differences we see between people are due to how their disease is affecting their brain. A major role is played by how the individual's personality and style, including how they communicated before, interact with the effects of the disease.

Communication makes use of a massive toolkit of skills and knowledge. Dementia may cause some tools to break, or even remove them from the kit entirely. But how this affects a person depends on how they used their toolkit in the first place. How good were they at tackling a new challenge, by using an old tool in a new way? We could say that, in a way, some people have been practising how to manage communication challenges for years, while others are less prepared. Just as a skilled craftsperson can improvise by adapting other tools when the tool they wanted isn't available, so a skilled communicator can often compensate for quite a while, despite living with a dementia. In turn, if communication difficulties are being handled well, in many ways the entire dementia will be less apparent and more manageable.

Language combines many different aspects of knowledge and ability. At the centre are the words we use. We're most aware of the words for things and ideas (nouns), for actions and processes (verbs), and for attributes and qualities (adjectives and adverbs). But there are also words that express relationships between ideas (such as *to*, *for*, *over*) or that help us specify certain detail in meaning (such when we choose to use *the* rather than *a*). As we'll see presently, word types have different characteristics when it comes to their susceptibility or resilience to dementia.

Words combine into phrases, clauses and sentences, and to make that happen we need the ability to hold the words in memory and put them together, using the patterns (grammar) specified in that particular language. We then need to get our vocal apparatus – or our hands, arms and face if we're using sign language, or our fingers if we're writing or typing – to produce the strings of sounds, signs or written letters that let us share the sentences with others.

To understand what others say to us, we have to unwrap streams of spoken material or signs, or decode written texts, in a manner that is more or less the reverse of what it takes to construct them. We'll see much more about all this in Chapter 3. For now, we'll just take a more general view of how dementias can interfere with those processes.

Problems with words and grammar

Perhaps the best-known problem people living with a dementia can have is finding specific words when they want them. For one reason or another, an idea just won't link itself to a word, or a word that they hear won't translate into a meaning. It's difficult to know if it's ever the case that the person actually doesn't know the word any more and will never produce it or understand it again. But that doesn't seem to be the typical situation. It's more likely that the word is still there somewhere, and it's just harder to find quickly using the searching methods that worked before.

Word-finding difficulties can affect us all at times. It can be inconvenient and sometimes even embarrassing when a word (particularly a name) escapes us. For people living with a dementia, it often won't take long for a missing word to create a problem, because they tend not to have as much confidence as other people that they can find a solution. Even if it takes only, say, ten extra seconds to find the word they want, that might be long enough for them to give up trying, or for someone else to chip in with what they *think* the person meant. Ten seconds could also be long enough for the person to lose the thread of what they wanted to say. If there's more than one other person present, the other two might just continue the conversation on their own. And if they change the topic, then by the time that missing word finally comes to mind, it'll be as useless as finally finding the Christmas decorations in February.

However, we all have various tricks to avoid a word-finding difficulty becoming too much of a problem. We've all ended up saying *you know* or *thingamajig* or *whatshisname* when a word or name wouldn't come to mind. These stand-in words let us get on with what we wanted to say. With luck, the other person will figure out who or what we meant, or we'll have chance to fill in the missing information later. Other solutions that we use are less obvious, and they might not be recognized for what they are. I'll say more about this in Chapter 5.

Depending on the type of dementia a person is dealing with, words can cause other types of difficulty too. People living with Alzheimer's, for example, sometimes come up with a word that's close in meaning but not the one they meant (e.g. *writing* for *reading*[2]), a word that seems to have little in common with the intended one (e.g. *dress* for *painting*) or a neologism – a word that doesn't exist at all (e.g. *ringlim*). In people living with semantic dementia (also known as fluent primary progressive aphasia), the form (i.e. the sound or spelling) of a word gets detached from its meaning. If you've ever tried learning a foreign language, you may recognize this experience. The teacher uses a word that you recognize. You know you're supposed to know it, but you just can't put a meaning to it. One example of the effect in semantic dementia comes from a British study published in the early 1990s: 'When asked, "Have you ever been to America?", she replied "What's America?", or asked,

---

2   The examples given here are from Heidi Hamilton's study of Elsie, a lady living with Alzheimer's disease (see Hamilton 2008, pp. 61–62).

"What's your favourite food?", she replied, "Food, food, I wish I knew what that was.'"[3]

Research has revealed other curious patterns as well. For example, people living with Alzheimer's seem to have greater difficulty naming animals and fruit than manmade items.[4] People living with nonfluent primary progressive aphasia seem to have more trouble coming up with verbs than nouns.[5] People living with semantic dementia struggle more with words for items that you can touch and see, than with words for abstract concepts like *love* and *importance*. Why these strange patterns exist is still debated, but it's a useful reminder that we shouldn't make hasty assumptions about what a person living with a dementia can and can't do – the difficulties can be quite specific (and also may not occur all the time).

When it comes to grammar, it's widely claimed that in most types of dementia there's little real change. In one of my own studies, Joan, a singing teacher who was living with Alzheimer's, did come up with a few odd sentences, such as 'That's very good because you've got attractive' and 'So that you've got that really feeling.'[6] But even in her case, her grammar was mostly okay, and the difficulties she experienced with language were largely because she couldn't find the words she needed. But if grammar isn't usually directly affected by dementia, that doesn't mean there can't be indirect effects. For example, if a person's dementia makes it hard for them to think quickly and hold information in memory while they construct what they want to say, it can look as if they have a problem with grammar. They might get halfway through the sentence and then tail off without finishing it. Or they might finish the sentence in a way that doesn't match how they started it. In other words, often the underlying problem is a more general one, such as a difficulty with memory, managing information or concentrating.

People living with Lewy body spectrum disorder can encounter communication difficulties because they can't provide much

---

3   Hodges et al. (1992, p. 1796)
4   Reilly, Troche and Grossman (2011)
5   Hillis, Oh and Ken (2004)
6   Wray (2010, p. 520)

information in what they say, or they get it out of order.[7] Some people living with fronto-temporal dementia become listless and unengaged, which means they have little to contribute to conversations. Others with fronto-temporal dementia have *reduced* inhibitions – perhaps because they've lost the ability to assess the situation they're in and what's expected of them. Still others become rather rigid in their thinking, and use a lot of repeated, stereotyped expressions, which limits the range of what they say.

Problems with meaning-making

The most powerful impact on communication doesn't come from difficulties with words or grammar. It comes from problems in sharing the *context* of a message. Context carries the broader elements of meaning. It gives us the information about why something was said, why it was said now and why it was said in a particular way. Context is the tool we use for filling in missing bits of information, and it helps us avoid getting the wrong end of the stick. As we'll see in Chapter 5, if communication is to work properly, the speaker needs to not only draw on the context as *they* see it, but also calculate how the *listener* will see the context. Unless they do this well, the listener simply won't respond in the way they hoped.

Context information is extremely vulnerable when someone's living with a dementia, for several reasons. The most important reason is that it depends on memory – memory for what's already happened and been said; memory for who people are and why they're there; and memory for how things happening *now* fit into what has, could and will take place at other times. People with memory impairments caused by dementia are likely to struggle to follow all that information. And even if a person living with a dementia doesn't have memory difficulties as such, they might find it hard to process the information fast enough to keep up. After all, the context is changing all the time.

---

7   Roberts and Orange (2013, p. 181)

Wider problems

So far, we've focused on difficulties with the process of communication itself. But that's not the end of the story. Many of the problems that people living with a dementia experience day by day come down to how they feel about themselves and others, and how others treat them. Even an apparently simple question or comment could leave them feeling uneasy or stressed. It's important that a dementia diagnosis isn't seen as a recipe for despair or rejection. Even when there are impairments to the communication tools, there's plenty that can still be done to get the best out of what remains.

ACTION POINTS FOR PEOPLE LIVING WITH A DEMENTIA

1. Try not to panic if you can't think of a word. Everyone experiences this problem sometimes. A good approach is to laugh, apologize and stop thinking about the word. It's likely to pop into your head in the end, all on its own.

2. It's quite likely that your dementia will sometimes cause you anxiety and stress. Make it your project to identify new approaches for handling these feelings. Here are some options you might consider: mindfulness; stroking your pet; going for a walk; playing a musical instrument or singing a favourite song; listening to music; weeding; watching a favourite film; rearranging flowers in a vase; sewing; knitting; drawing; painting; craftwork; puzzle books; colouring in. If you're not sure what will help, ask your doctor or a friend or family member to suggest some stress-reducing activities.

3. It can be embarrassing and upsetting to forget someone's name. But it's just a name, after all. Reassure the person that you still know who they are. If you're not sure who they are, then it's usually better to just ask them.

4. If you're having problems with your language, tell people. If they know, then you don't need to hide the difficulties, and they can be more understanding.

5. Are you the kind of person who hates it when other people complete your sentence for you? Or are you grateful? Or does it depend on the situation? The people you talk with may not know how you feel and what you want, so why not politely tell them?

6. If you're worried about getting into situations where you can't express yourself well enough, why not write down what you want to say (or get someone else to)? You can keep a note with you, in your pocket or stored on your phone. By planning in advance you'll be confident that you have the words there. You can read them out, or hand your note to the other person to read for themselves.

7. If you don't always understand what people say to you, remember this: they do want you to understand, because otherwise they're wasting their breath! So, ask them to speak more slowly or say something again. Try to keep cheerful and not be stressed. That way, they won't be stressed either and they'll be happy to help you.

ACTION POINTS FOR FAMILIES, FRIENDS AND PROFESSIONALS

1. If you're feeling frustrated as you communicate with a person living with a dementia, remember that they're feeling even more frustrated than you are. They need your kindness and support not your tuts and pouts.

2. If you're not sure whether to chip in with a word that the person's struggling to find, ask them if they'd like your help or not. Don't assume they'll always give the same answer, because it may depend on what they're talking about, where they are or how they feel about the topic. For example, it might mean a great deal to them to recall the name of a grandchild on their own.[8]

---

8   Richard Taylor (2007, p. 192), living with Alzheimer's, makes this comment about not being able to recall the names of his grandchildren or his daughter-in-law: 'I want to know that I know their names, and if it takes me a few extra seconds to find the names, please just stand around and wait with me until the correct answer comes out through my mouth.'

3. To help you understand the challenges with language that the person living with the dementia is experiencing, think about situations you've been in that are similar in some way. Perhaps you were trying to use a foreign language, or you were very tired, or you were so intimidated by the situation that it made you tongue-tied. How did you want others to support you?

4. Keep in mind that tiredness increases the risk of stress and of communication difficulties. Become aware of how the time of day and people's sleep patterns (including yours) can affect situations.

5. Take an interest in the patterns you notice in the language difficulties of the person you interact with. Observing and being curious about things can help you keep emotional distance, so you don't make the problem worse.

6. If the person living with the dementia doesn't understand what you say to them, try not to show frustration or annoyance – it's not their fault. Have another go. There are plenty of skills you can gradually develop for expressing messages in other ways, including using gestures, pictures, and so on.

ACTION POINTS FOR BYSTANDERS

1. If you encounter a person who seems a little confused or who's having difficulty communicating, you have a choice: help and support them, or walk away. What would you want someone to do if it were you or someone you care about?

2. In many ways, 'bystanders', who don't have to engage day-on-day with people living with a dementia, can be a very important source of support. They don't come into the situation with lots of assumptions about what the person can and can't do, and they don't tend to second guess things on their behalf. It will often be a chance encounter with an outsider that lightens up the day of a person living with a dementia and/or their close family carer. You can make a big difference even with small kindnesses.

CHAPTER TWO

The Things We Can and Can't Control about Dementia

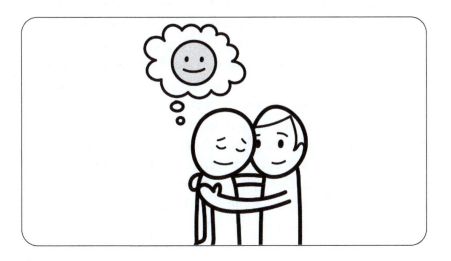

Joan

Joan (not her real name), a renowned professional opera singer, taught singing after she retired from the stage. In her mid-80s, she was still teaching, despite marked symptoms of Alzheimer's disease. It's quite unusual for people living with a dementia to still be working in their 80s, but freelance musicians often don't get around to retiring. Over the years, the Alzheimer's had no doubt just crept up on her. For as long as it didn't prevent her doing what she loved, why would she stop?

One weekend, Joan arrived at a study centre to teach workshops for amateur singers.[1] Each of the nine singers on the course had prepared three or four solo songs to sing to Joan and the others. Joan's job was to listen to each person in turn, giving them equal time and opportunity to sing, and provide feedback on how to improve. She had to advise them, as necessary, on their breathing, vocal production, diction, pronunciation of English, French, German or Italian, and interpretation. On the Sunday afternoon, an informal concert would allow the participants to perform to each other and to locals who often came in to listen.

It was fairly evident to me that Joan was living with Alzheimer's. She had severe difficulties finding words and often couldn't follow what people said in general conversation. At meals, she was either hesitant, letting others speak up for her, or else dominated the conversation with statements that seemed out of place for the situation.

Yet in the music room, teaching the students, things were very different. She worked with confidence, focus, energy and dignity. If she couldn't find a word, she sang the phrase to demonstrate what she wanted, or mimed an action to show, for example, that she wanted the singer to put more energy into the phrase. She provided enough information for the singers to figure out what she probably meant, and she used a wealth of techniques to fulfil her teacher role.

Without question, having this authority and knowledge played a huge part in how well she communicated. It gave her confidence, credibility and a strong sense of identity. The students were keen to support her as she tried to express herself, because they wanted to learn. It was a social environment that worked exceptionally well for everyone.

An important positive influence was the piano accompanist, David. He was a singing teacher in his own right, and could easily have just taken over from her, if he'd wished. But instead, with remarkable sensitivity and skill, he deftly supported Joan in her role. If he noticed that a singer hadn't quite understood what Joan meant, he would wait a second and then say something like, 'So, if you do as Joan said,

---

1   For more on Joan, see Wray (2010, 2020b).

and hold that note on longer then...' In this way, he restated what he believed Joan meant, but without giving any hint that she'd been unsuccessful in conveying it herself. David was the glue that held things together, but he let Joan's ideas continue to be the substance of the classes, so there was no doubt who the teacher was.

That weekend of workshops was an unusual and extreme example of how someone living with Alzheimer's can communicate. But it demonstrates the impact that a positive social environment can have, not only on a person living with a dementia but also on those around them. This chapter examines the ways in which we can all contribute to building and sustaining such positive environments.

Getting dementia – a roll of the dice?

Life happens. Few of us will escape illness or disability at some point in our life. But let's not beat about the bush. Dementia is a tough illness to get. As yet there's no cure. The few available treatments only slow down the progression of the symptoms and reduce their impact a little. So far, nothing can stop dementia, or reverse it. When more is understood about dementia-causing diseases, we can hope for a considerable improvement in the outlook. In the meantime, we can all do our part by participating in research that looks for cures and better treatments.

It may seem that getting dementia is like getting struck by lightning – we don't know who'll get it, and it's just bad luck. That's true to an extent, but, as a chess player might say to a mountaineer, not everyone has an equal chance of getting struck by lightning! It's true that some aspects of our vulnerability to dementia are beyond our control. But there are definitely things we can do, both to reduce our chances of getting dementia and, if we already have a diagnosis, to hold the symptoms at bay.

In this chapter we'll examine *reserve*, or resistance, to dementia. The amount of reserve we have shapes when and to what extent a dementia-causing disease will have real impact on our daily life. I'll describe four types of reserve. Two of them are well established in the research literature. *Brain reserve* is the ability of the brain's structure to withstand the damage caused by brain diseases. *Cognitive reserve* is the brain's capacity to continue functioning despite physical damage. The other two types of reserve – *social* and *emotional* – are my own idea. They're a way to capture how people's environment and internal emotional resources can shape their life with a dementia.

Brain reserve

A paper published in the February 1988 issue of *Annals of Neurology* sparked awareness of brain reserve.[2] A team of US scientists and clinicians headed by Robert Katzman examined the brains of 137 deceased individuals of average age 85. Some hadn't had any symptoms of dementia during their life, yet their brains had almost as much of the damage associated with Alzheimer's disease as people with significant dementia. In other words, their brains had the disease, but their cognitive function hadn't been affected. Why didn't these people have symptoms of dementia? What was special about them? They had heavier brains and more large neurons (nerve cells in the brain) than average, and the researchers concluded that this had given them some ability to resist the effects of the disease.

Later research revealed that larger brains, with more neural connections, are better at absorbing the damage caused by disease. This allows the brain to continue functioning relatively normally. As a result, the person can continue their life without any obvious symptoms. This characteristic became known as *brain reserve* or *neural reserve*. We can think of our brain connectivity as a bit like a road system. If there are lots of roads, and they're wide, then even if one road gets partly or completely blocked, it won't be difficult to find alternative routes to our destination.

Just what decides how much brain reserve someone has isn't fully known, but it may include our genetic inheritance and/or how we develop in the womb.[3] The size of someone's skull seems to predict brain reserve[4] – large brains need a larger skull, after all. But our brain

---

2   Katzman et al. (1988)
3   Bartrés-Faz and Arenaza-Urquijo (2011); Deters et al. (2017)
4   Graves et al. (1996); Perneczky et al. (2010)

also changes throughout our life, and it's possible that people vary in how efficient and flexible their brains are. This could affect how a brain first grows and connects up and also how easily alternative brain areas can become involved, if the usual ones are damaged or overstretched.[5]

Cognitive reserve

Cognitive reserve is the ability to take advantage of the brain's structures to achieve things. If brain reserve is like a well-connected road system, then cognitive reserve is how you use that system. If you want to get the benefit of a large and complex road network, it helps to have a fast and reliable car and to know your way around, with different options for getting from A to B. Someone with high cognitive reserve is agile in their thinking, and able to work things through and figure out different possible solutions to challenges.

Cognitive reserve is important because dementia-causing diseases often damage the cells or connections we've always used to achieve certain tasks. It's the equivalent of an accident leading to the closure of a road on our usual route to the supermarket. If we come to a roadblock, we'll need another route. If the road network is good, there will be alternatives. But our ability to get to the supermarket will depend on how familiar we are with those roads. A driver who often experiments with different routes or has visited a lot of places will find it relatively easy to navigate a new way to the destination. And, importantly, a driver like that will also have lots of confidence that a way can be found. In contrast, a driver who never strays off the most familiar routes from A to B could be flummoxed by a roadblock, have little idea which way to go and feel nervous about trying.

The same seems to apply when it comes to using our brains. People who've explored many ideas and skills, who are used to thinking around an issue or task in different ways and who are confident doing so seem to be more resilient to dementia symptoms. If their brain becomes damaged by one of the dementia-causing diseases, so they

---

5   Stern et al. (2008)

can't use routes in their brain network as they used to, they simply find alternatives. Probably for this reason, people's level of cognitive reserve is thought to be closely linked to how much education they've had. Education gets a person to look at things in different ways, and so it's good brain training and builds cognitive reserve. Having said that, students can sit in a classroom without learning much. And some people will have increased their cognitive reserve throughout their lives despite having left school at a young age. Therefore, it's not really safe to predict someone's cognitive reserve, or their risk of dementia, based only on when they left school. Each case needs to be looked at individually.

Aside from formal education, various activities get promoted as helpful for boosting cognitive reserve. For example, it's often claimed that doing crossword puzzles and sudoku can reduce dementia risk. In fact, the research evidence is rather mixed on this issue. It's true that people who enjoy such activities tend to be in the group that staves off dementia symptoms for longer. But it's difficult for researchers to separate out why. It might not be that the puzzles themselves are building cognitive reserve. Perhaps these people already have high cognitive reserve for another reason, with one side-effect being that they've developed confidence in language and maths, which would make the puzzles more enjoyable than they are for someone with lower cognitive reserve.

If 'brain-training' activities do improve people's ability to deal with dementia symptoms, taking them up late in life might not work, unfortunately. According to one recent study,[6] cognitively challenging activities did have a protective effect, but it was built up over many years. You need to have been doing these activities all your life. Having said that, as the researchers in that study point out, it's certainly not *harmful* to take up cognitively based pastimes later in life. Meanwhile, people who've used their brains in their daily life for many years may, in retirement, need to look for new activities that are cognitively stimulating, so they don't lose the benefits they've built up over the years. Finally, there are indirect benefits to activities

---

6   Staff et al. (2018)

that challenge the brain. Many studies indicate that keeping our mind busy helps combat depression. And keeping depression at bay is helpful in its own right in reducing the risk of dementia.[7]

So, it seems that cognitive reserve arises from lifelong habits. Two in particular have drawn the interest of researchers. One is playing a musical instrument,[8] which involves a number of abilities used together, including physical skill, reading music, counting and artistic interpretation. It often has the additional advantage of being a sociable activity, which is good for people's general mental health.

The other lifelong behaviour that might be protective against dementia symptoms is the regular use of two languages. This effect has been found in bilingual communities in several countries, including Canada,[9] the USA,[10] Wales,[11] Italy[12] and India.[13] Typically, the advantage is measured in terms of how many years older bilinguals are than monolinguals when they first go to a memory clinic with early dementia symptoms. The average effect seems to be around four years of extra life before the symptoms show. It doesn't mean that the bilinguals develop dementia-causing *diseases* any later. Rather, they can live with the disease without any problems for longer. However, critics[14] have challenged the quality of the research evidence for these effects, which leaves it unclear for now whether the advantage is real.

Social reserve

So far, we've reviewed two types of reserve. Brain reserve is the level of protection people have against the brain damage arising from dementia-causing diseases. Cognitive reserve plays a role in determining when dementia symptoms appear in those who have developed these diseases. Now we turn to another type of reserve.

---

7 Livingston et al. (2017)
8 Balbag, Pedersen and Gatz (2014); Gaser and Schlaug (2003); Hudziak et al. (2014); Hyde et al. (2009)
9 Bialystok, Craik and Freedman (2007); Chertkow et al. (2010)
10 Gollan et al. (2011)
11 Clare et al. (2016)
12 Perani et al. (2017)
13 Alladi et al. (2013)
14 For example, Baum and Titone (2014); de Bot (2017); Morton (2014); Mukadam, Sommerlad and Livingston (2017); Paap and Greenberg (2013); Valian (2015)

Social reserve is a concept that I developed as I tried to understand what *else* makes a difference to how quickly people living with a dementia-causing disease become badly affected by the symptoms.

In my book *The Dynamics of Dementia Communication*, I define social reserve as 'the currency of resilience located in a person's cultural and social context, both local and global'.[15] What this means is that we gain, or fail to gain, protective benefits according to the situations we find ourselves in and the people we find ourselves with. Unlike brain reserve and cognitive reserve, which are fundamentally *within* the individual, social reserve is built primarily *outside* the individual. Even though people can do things to build their own social reserve, it's largely up to society as a whole to create social reserve. In other words, we need to build it for each other. Building social reserve is within our gift as a society and as individuals, and it's something that we should all be thinking about trying to support.

Social reserve protects all of us from unkindness, thoughtlessness and inconvenience. And it's a buffer against a variety of factors that affect the severity of dementia, including depression, loneliness, frustration, uncaring people and unnecessary medication. Four subtypes of social reserve can be separated out, though they connect up to quite an extent. They are: *infrastructure, attitudes, social groups* and *social credibility*, and they're described in the sections that follow. With high levels of these four types of social reserve, people living with a dementia are less likely to feel abandoned, discriminated against or ignored, and they'll thrive in a supportive environment that lets them use their remaining abilities and live as well as possible. As we'll see, it's not only people living with a dementia themselves who benefit from high social reserve. Their families and carers also need it.

Social and health infrastructure

One of the most distressing and challenging experiences for people living with a dementia and their family members is fighting with the system that's supposed to support them. Infrastructure is the

---

15   Wray (2020b, p. 76)

set of arrangements that society sets up to help people navigate the complexities of their lives. It includes primary medical services, hospital, respite and residential care, public transport, access to legal rights, information, communications (including post, telephone and internet), media (including newspapers, radio, television, streaming and social media), advice, financial support, signage, the design of streets and buildings, and so on.

As one person living with a dementia said about getting her diagnosis, 'Nobody offers help, you've got to go and find it and ask for it'.[16] Not being able to get basic information, not knowing where advice or help can be found and not knowing who to inform to get the right support can all quickly wear people down. When infrastructure is inadequate or isn't properly coordinated, it can take hours to achieve even basic things – on the phone trying to reach the right person, or trekking from office to office to make sure that different providers (e.g. care companies and health workers) each know what the other is doing. The structuring of agencies and services in many countries takes too little account of the needs of people living with a dementia, who might, for example, struggle to follow telephone instructions to *press one* for this and *two* for that.

So, what determines how good the infrastructure is? Typically, when infrastructure is poor, the finger is pointed at financial strains on public services. When, year by year, more has to be done with less, it's inevitable that provision will be less complete and effective, and less joined up. There won't be staff available to 'go the extra mile' of ensuring cases are followed up and cross-referenced with other providers. We can blame the politicians, but politicians are voted in by the people. That means it's a public choice to deprioritize good infrastructure. It's up to all of us to think hard about whether it's worth having low taxes if it means we don't have the core services we all might need. If we're to understand why infrastructure is not better, we need to think about our attitudes, including our attitudes towards dementia itself.

---

16   Smith et al. (2019, p. 8)

Attitudes

What happens when people discover that a friend or colleague has a dementia diagnosis? What happens when, in a general hospital, the staff are informed that their newest arrival on the ward not only has a broken hip but also dementia? What assumptions and beliefs are triggered, and how do they affect attitudes and expectations? What behaviour will the person living with dementia experience from others? If they're a bit drowsy, say, will that be interpreted as confusion due to dementia? If they're grumpy, will that be interpreted as a symptom of dementia, rather than something that could be attended to?

In hospitals, as also in care homes, staff may be quick to use medication to deal with any anger or frustration in people living with a dementia, rather than delving into what's troubling them. Yet medication is often unnecessary. In one research study, medication was routinely used in a residential home to manage 'difficult' behaviours in people living with a dementia. When changes were made in the approach to care, it was possible to reduce the use of antipsychotic drugs to zero, with no increased problems. Indeed, the researcher reports that 'people who came into the unit often commented on how alert and contented everyone looked. In addition, the residents were more cooperative, and interested in what was going on around them.'[17]

Those who haven't been specifically trained in communicating with people living with a dementia are often strongly influenced by what they've picked up over the years from the news, social media, anecdotes, jokes and depictions in books, films, TV, and so on. Where dementia is presented negatively, it will shape the choices people make. Neighbours and friends might keep their distance, anxious about getting into an embarrassing situation or about being drawn into some sort of obligation they feel they can't keep up. They might feel that they don't know what to say or do and that life will just be a lot easier if they cut the person out of their social circle as much as possible. Although this might sound selfish, it's also understandable,

---

17   O'Sullivan (2011, p. 116)

since most people have their own daily challenges to deal with, and additional uncertainty is not likely to be welcome. The solution is to reduce that uncertainty by giving people more information and a more positive presentation of what people living with a dementia are like and are able to do.

When others keep their distance from people living with a dementia, it can make it more difficult for them to adjust to their diagnosis and the various challenges of their daily life. Their own attitudes and beliefs, built up over the years, may not help, and now they might also feel nervous about asking people for assistance, in case the response is lukewarm. Simple matters like asking a neighbour to check the electricity meter reading or give them a lift to an appointment could seem too emotionally risky. As a result, quite small things that would be easily fixed can get in the way of living well. And the same issues can arise for family members caring for a person living with a dementia. They too may feel avoided and ignored. They too may be nervous of reaching out for assistance in case they're turned down. Social reserve is a commodity that they also need.

Fortunately, things are changing, albeit slowly. There's more emphasis on 'dementia awareness' and inclusivity. Environments are made more 'dementia friendly', and basic training is available for ordinary people to learn more about the symptoms of dementia and how to support people dealing with them. Simply realizing that the reason a person is taking extra time in the supermarket queue, asking a question more than once or struggling to take in information is because they're doing their best while living with a dementia can immediately make us more tolerant and supportive. But more still needs to be done if basic attitudes are to be altered. Exciting new initiatives include bringing young children into regular contact with people living with a dementia. Children are very accepting and older people love to engage with them, and even teach and guide them. The positive attitudes that this sort of experience can instil in the young are a great investment for the future.

Another effective way to change behaviours and attitudes towards dementia is through the many different media we have daily exposure to. There are now some excellent novels, feature films and documentaries about people living with a dementia. But there are still plenty of depictions that are negative caricatures. News reports still often focus on the horrors of poor care more than the success stories of good care and support.

Social groups

So far, social reserve has been described as something that a person living with a dementia or a family supporter must simply hope is available and positive. But when it comes to social groups, they can do more for themselves. It goes without saying that someone surrounded by truly supportive family, friends and neighbours is likely to have a more positive experience than someone trying to cope alone. Loneliness is a major risk both for people with a dementia diagnosis and for those supporting them. Families are often geographically separated. A person living with a dementia may not have any relative near enough to help on a daily basis. People who've lived privately in the past might not have a network of friends, and it's common these days for us not to know our neighbours. People can, however, still do something for themselves, such as joining clubs and groups, attending a place of worship, and so on. Of course, it's important for the members of such groups to be welcoming, and to recognize how vulnerable people living with a dementia can be.

There are lots of advantages to spending time with other people. We benefit from eye contact, physical touch, humour and conversation.[18] Socializing gives us a reason to focus on others, which helps us keep perspective and take an interest in the world. But, as with the other types of social reserve, it's vital that the people who *aren't* affected by dementia create and maintain positive experiences for those who are, so they can gain full benefit from social groups.

---

18   Livingston et al. (2017, p. 31)

Social credibility

The general attitudes and assumptions about dementia in the community can mean that people living with a dementia lose their 'voice'. That is, their preferences and priorities are ignored, while other people tell them what's best for them. Richard Taylor, a person living with Alzheimer's who wrote insightfully and movingly about his experiences, noticed how people often ignored him and talked to the person he was with.[19] He also felt sad that 'People are no longer dependent on me to do something for them, I am dependent on them'.[20] Family and friends may need gentle reminders that their best intentions can be misplaced. In one study, an older woman living with a dementia said:

> I still want some control over my affairs and how things are done… The kids are more inclined to tell me what I should be doing. And sometimes I don't take their advice after thinking it through, and they have had to learn that's ok too… If you're dealing with older people, let them make the decisions instead of forcing things.[21]

Keeping some ability to make their own decisions is important for people's confidence and self-respect, at a time when they may be full of doubts and anxieties, and perhaps tempted to believe that others know best. As the neuropsychologist and dementia specialist Steven Sabat points out, 'To see oneself, and to be seen by others, principally in terms of what one cannot do, cannot but weaken one's sense of self-worth, or self-esteem, and increase one's sense of being burdensome and deficient.'[22]

The line is difficult to draw. It's certainly true that some forms of dementia weaken a person's judgement. And problems with memory and cognitive processing could mean that the person doesn't have all the facts. Nevertheless, a dementia diagnosis doesn't suddenly remove people's desire to make decisions about their own lives, or their ability to do so.

---

19   Taylor (2007, p. 152)
20   Taylor (2007, p. 127)
21   Smith et al. (2019, p. 43)
22   Sabat (2001, p. 118)

Allowing a person with a developing cognitive impairment to remain centrally involved in their own decision-making is not always easy, either in practical terms or emotionally. If a family member or professional firmly believes one course of action is best, and the person living with the dementia doesn't agree, it can become a battle of wills that's wearing and distressing for everyone. But it'll certainly help if the desires of the person living with the dementia are taken seriously and they're allowed to contribute to discussions and the final decision. If something does have to be decided against the person's will (e.g. significant alterations in how or where they're cared for), then it will help to find opportunities for them to be involved in some aspects of the changes. For example, if they must move to a residential home, let them look at webpages or brochures to help decide which one. And let them have a say in which of their possessions they take with them.

Shaping social reserve

The four subtypes of social reserve interact with each other. Policies are shaped by public attitudes. Attitudes are shaped by, as well as reflected in, the media. The willingness of individuals to welcome people living with a dementia into their social circles is also shaped by society's attitudes. If people living with a dementia aren't given a chance, and treated as able to participate, they'll become anxious and may withdraw from social settings, making it more difficult for others to reach and support them. How people think about dementia isn't just a result of their own observation and experience. Cultures carry longstanding, often unspoken, patterns of belief and behaviour towards, for example, ageing, disability and illness. These patterns shape the ways we view our world.

As we'll see in Chapter 4, dementia, and particularly memory loss, challenges people's deep-seated understandings of their identity. In many societies, people define who they are in terms of what they've done in their lives. If they can't recall that information, it can make them feel that they're disappearing. And those around them may struggle to build a relationship with them without access to their life story.

Building up social reserve is no easy matter. We need to chip away at the underlying currents of belief and assumption. One way is to help people learn, through experience, just how fulfilling it can be to interact with a person living with a dementia.

Emotional reserve

How well do people living with a dementia and their close relatives cope with the practical impact of the disease? Some people are cast into deep despair, while others seem to manage the challenges more easily. Part of the difference between these people may be their level of *emotional reserve*, which, like social reserve, is a concept that emerged for me in the course of my research into the broad experience of communicating in the dementia context.[23]

Emotional reserve is the personal capacity to handle misfortune without losing too much confidence or sense of identity. Living with a dementia may bring emotions to the surface that have been kept under control in the past, and it may cause new, deep feelings of anxiety. Meanwhile those supporting people living with a dementia are also likely to experience additional emotional strain.

Having high emotional reserve makes it possible to stay in touch with our feelings, so we notice what's happening. It helps us avoid automatic emotional responses, so we can reflect on the options we have available. People with high emotional reserve can continue to recognize and value the many aspects of their life that are not shaped by their dementia. They stop the dementia taking over their entire identity. They avoid becoming *just* a person living with a dementia, or *just* the daily supporter of one, and continue to be a person, a parent, a grandparent, a friend, with all the associated pleasures and responsibilities. As a result, they can more easily keep a positive approach to living well. We're all different and some people are naturally more emotionally resilient than others,[24] but that doesn't mean we can't all build up our resilience to some extent.

Not surprisingly, our emotional reserve is strongly shaped by

---

23   Wray (2020b)
24   See Kitwood (1997, pp. 72–73) for discussion of this.

the level of social reserve we can access. If people around us are pleasant and supportive, we'll feel better and more able to cope. If the infrastructure works well, so we can get information and assistance easily, we'll be less stressed. This applies both to people living with a dementia and to those who support them. Importantly, professional carers and family members who have high emotional reserve are in a strong position to act with wisdom and kindness. As a result, they can help people living with a dementia build up their own emotional reserve. In contrast, when carers and family have, themselves, only low emotional reserve, then frustration, annoyance and hurtful interaction are likely to follow, as everyone tries to deal with their bruised feelings.

So, where does emotional reserve come from? Mostly, it comes from emotional intelligence, which is a more stable aspect of someone's personality, whereas emotional reserve will ebb and flow according to the situation. Some people are just naturally calmer and more 'together' than others. But we also develop greater or lesser levels of emotional maturity from our life experiences, from our personal beliefs or philosophy, by watching how others respond to challenges and from the general attitudes in our culture about how we can and might behave.

Figure 2.1 shows how helpful it is to develop ways of increasing our emotional reserve even if we're under emotional pressure ourselves. When two people have, between them, enough emotional reserve to cope with the pressures of a situation, they should come through without too many problems. But if one person has a lower level of emotional reserve than is needed, then not all of the emotional pressures can be absorbed jointly. That's when tensions are likely to bubble up. If one person can increase their emotional reserve to manage more of the pressure, then they can prevent difficulties arising so easily.

It won't always be the person living with the dementia whose emotional resilience flags first. However, if it's a family member who's finding it difficult to cope with the additional emotional pressures, it may be asking a lot to expect the person living with the dementia to pick up the slack.

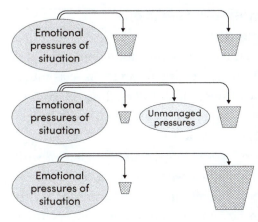

Figure 2.1: The benefit of increased emotional reserve

In practice, it's inevitable that sometimes we'll find ourselves in the situation depicted in the middle layer of Figure 2.1, where not all the emotional pressures can be absorbed and managed. The psychiatrist Bere Miesen offers useful advice to carers on how to neutralize emotional tension (focusing, in this instance, on signs of aggression). He suggests thinking about what's happened to create it:

> The process of trying to understand 'why', often provides carers with possible handles to prevent aggression. In this way, the person with dementia will not be 'written off' as an 'unappreciative stranger'. Also, the carer is less likely to blame themselves for the aggressive behaviour of the person with dementia. Feelings of uncertainty and guilt will be reduced (*It must be my fault!*). Hopefully this will allow a carer to continue to think of the person with dementia as being likeable, kind, or sympathetic.[25]

What Miesen illustrates here is how kindness and curiosity pave the way to building additional emotional reserve – situations that seemed too difficult to deal with become more easily manageable.

---

25 Miesen (1999, p. 210)

Building social and emotional reserve through good communication

It's in everyone's interests that people living with a dementia, and also their close family and their professional carers, have as much social and emotional reserve as possible. It's like oiling the cogs of a big machine – things will run more smoothly and life will be less jarring and uncomfortable for everyone.

Building social reserve is everyone's responsibility. It begins with individual personal actions that we take when we encounter a person living with a dementia within our family, in the community or as part of our job. It includes face-to-face encounters, phone conversations and written communications, whether letters, emails or social media messages. It extends also to the choices we make in local and national elections, because they shape policy decisions about the quality of the infrastructure in our health, social and transport systems. We can also speak up when the media present negative impressions of people living with a dementia and their family supporters. And we can lend our voice to campaigns and initiatives that make our world more inclusive.

We can offer our skills and time to give practical help to those who are intimidated by modern technology but need to use it to get things done. We can just bite the bullet and go and have a conversation with someone living with a dementia, even though we know that it might become awkward if, for example, they don't recall who we are, or what they previously told us. We can model the level of care and attention that we want for everyone living with a dementia on what we'd want for our own mum or dad, grandma or grandpa, spouse, neighbour or friend.

When we build others' social reserve, it helps them increase their emotional reserve, making them more resilient to the inevitable ups and downs of daily life. At the heart of such acts of kindness and solidarity towards each other is good communication. And the effectiveness of communication can be improved by understanding how it works. What drives us to communicate? What determines the choices we make about what we say versus what we leave unsaid? What shapes the expression of our messages? Why do the things we say sometimes get misinterpreted, or taken the wrong way? The rest of this book delves into these questions.

ACTION POINTS FOR PEOPLE LIVING WITH A DEMENTIA

1. Why not volunteer to participate in research into dementia?[26] It might not lead to discoveries that help you directly, but it could help people in the future, including your own younger family members. It means you would be making a difference and giving something back to society – something you can only give because of your dementia.
2. Look for opportunities to join groups and get to know people. Take an interest in others and it will give you many benefits, including their interest in you.
3. Be prepared to speak up for yourself if others are taking over your affairs. Ask them to explain why they have their view. Ask them to help you feed into decisions about your life so that what's decided is acceptable to you as well as others.
4. Start noticing how you, and others, respond emotionally in different situations – for example, when an object gets broken, or dinner is late, or someone comes to the house. Can you tell what sparks frustration, annoyance or sadness? Sometimes, it's not what happens, but what someone says or does as a result. Noticing is the first step to having choice about what to do.

ACTION POINTS FOR FAMILIES, FRIENDS AND PROFESSIONALS

1. Volunteer as a participant in research.[27] There's a particular need for family members of people with a dementia diagnosis,

---

26 One route into volunteering is here: www.joindementiaresearch.nihr.ac.uk/content/volunteersheet

27 One route into volunteering is here: www.joindementiaresearch.nihr.ac.uk/content/volunteersheet

so that the hereditary aspects of the dementia-causing diseases can be better understood.

2. Join groups, so you have a wider network of friends and supporters. Consider groups for people such as yourself, caring for someone living with a dementia, but also groups that can bring out other aspects of your identity and interests.

3. In your eagerness to fix new and difficult situations, be careful not to take decisions out of the hands of the person living with the dementia. They may already feel insecure and anxious. Giving them opportunities to make decisions will help build their emotional reserve. If you feel you have to overrule them, look for opportunities to let them make other, smaller, decisions that will cushion the impact of the big one.

4. Notice how you, and those around you, respond emotionally to different situations, and what seems to spark frustration, annoyance or sadness. Noticing is the first step to having choices.

5. Read *Alzheimer's from the Inside Out* by Richard Taylor. It's a deeply moving account by a person living with Alzheimer's, about his daily feelings and experiences. It may give you insights into what can help or hinder good communication and relationships.

ACTION POINTS FOR BYSTANDERS

1. Volunteer as a participant in research.[28] Projects need 'control' participants, who are not affected by a dementia themselves and may or may not have family members who are.

2. Lobby for improved infrastructure and make any changes you can in your own daily environment, to help people living with a dementia have a good experience when they encounter you or the services you provide.

3. Be supportive of people living with a dementia and their family carers if they join your group or club. Just turning up may have

---

28 One route into volunteering is here: www.joindementiaresearch.nihr.ac.uk/content/ volunteersheet

been a major achievement for them. The benefits of attending may be substantial, so they need encouragement and support in continuing. Be tolerant if a person living with a dementia takes time to settle or can't recall who people are, or what the group's customs and practices are.

4. Be aware of the dividing line between helping someone and doing things for them. Unless the person asks you to take over, try to support them in doing things for themselves.

5. Notice how you respond emotionally when you are interacting with people living with a dementia. Also look for indications of their own emotions. Draw on your experience from other aspects of your life to think about what choices you have, as you seek to be as kind and supportive as possible.

CHAPTER THREE

Why We Communicate

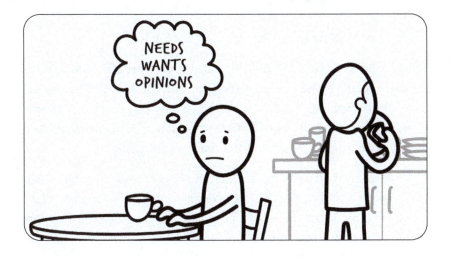

Bill and Danuta

The following conversation comes from Danuta Lipinska's book *Person-centred Counselling for People with Dementia*.[1] The book shows how counselling techniques can help people living with a dementia speak for themselves, resolve emotional issues and learn new ways to manage their symptoms. In the run-up to this excerpt, Danuta explains to the reader that saying something over and over again can mean it has some particular significance for the person. And that's what her conversation with Bill reveals:[2]

---

1   Lipinska (2009)
2   Lipinska (2009, p. 98)

Danuta: You're wondering if we have been down this road before, aren't you Bill?

Bill: Yeah.

Danuta: Yes Bill, you have told me about your boss before, but if you feel you'd like to tell me again that's OK. [Pause. Bill looking anxiously around and fidgeting with his fingers] You seem a bit worried?

Bill: Just seems important to tell you.

Danuta: I'm wondering if there's something you are trying to get at, and I'm missing it?

Bill: Yeah.

Danuta: Shall we see where we go with it Bill?

Lipinska notes in her commentary that each time Bill talked of his boss, the events he described were different, but the theme was the same – bullying. She wanted to pin down why this particular theme was being triggered so often. As the conversation continued, Bill told her a story about his boss[3] and the reason emerged:

Danuta: You're feeling stupid and that's kind of embarrassing? When your boss would get mad at you in front of your friends? [He's nodding, but not moving] Like maybe how it is when your memory doesn't work like you want it to?

Bill: Yeah. [BIG sigh]

Danuta: That's a big sigh Bill, from way down deep. [I sigh like he did] It feels like here... [I put my fist in my gut]

Bill: [Looks right at me and straightens a little] That's right.

Danuta: [Nodding slowly] Right. [Silence] I think I get what you want to say Bill. Can I try and say it back to you?

Bill: Yeah, OK.

Danuta: OK. Stop me if I get it wrong or go too fast. The feeling you get when your memory doesn't work is like how you felt around your boss when he was mad at you?

Bill: [Nodding]

Danuta: You feel stupid, embarrassed?

---

3   Lipinska (2009, pp. 99–100)

> *Bill: Yep. [Moving now, changing position but still making himself small in the chair]*
> *Danuta: Is it like shame?*
> *Bill: [Looking down and away] Yes, that's it. Shame. I feel ashamed.*
> *Danuta: [Nodding] Mmmm.*
> *Bill: Stupid and ashamed. I can't do anything about it.*

This conversation is interesting for a number of reasons. First, we see how expertly Danuta enables Bill to express his feelings and ideas. She uses several techniques, such as giving him time and space to think and speak and indicating that she's fully engaged with his agendas. She offers suggestions about what he might want to say. Yet she's careful to give him control, by inviting him to tell her if she's right or not. (We'll see a similar technique in operation in Chapter 9.)

Second, she's tolerant when Bill wants to talk about his boss again. She doesn't suggest that since she's heard it before he can save his breath. She's not annoyed or frustrated. Instead, she lets him talk about whatever he wants to, and she guesses that there may be a reason why he's continuing to raise the topic. It turns out she's right. There's a deep emotional link between the bullying he experienced at work and how he feels now as he deals with his dementia. Perhaps he can more easily point to these feelings in this indirect way. Or perhaps he can't fully distinguish between the events in his mind. Either way, because Danuta gives him space to say what he needs to, she's able to pick up on a major issue that he might not otherwise have expressed. What she does here so expertly is read between the lines. As we'll see in this chapter, that's one of the core elements of effective communication.

Third, note how both Bill and Danuta use non-verbal signals as well as language – through the way they sit, the sighs, nods and *mmms* they make, and the silences. These remind us that communication isn't just about words.

Another thing we learn from the conversation is that Bill is *worried* about repeating himself. It's often tempting to assume that when people living with a dementia say the same things more than once, they don't know they're doing so. But that's not necessarily the case.

There are many examples of people living with a dementia being aware of their tendency to repeat themselves. They might say, *as I said before*[4] or add *again* when asking a question for a second time, as in *what's your name again?*.[5]

Even if a person doesn't recall that they previously said something, they'll soon realize something's wrong if they see people roll their eyes or glaze over. And if the other person says *yes, I already know that*, or *I already answered that question three times,* they'll surely experience some sort of negative reaction. They could be confused, if they're not sure what exactly they have said before and what they haven't. They might feel ashamed for boring or annoying the other person, even though it's not their fault. And they might feel anxious, if their strong urge to tell their story or ask their question conflicts with another desire – to avoid getting a negative response from the other person. It would be so easy for them to decide not to bother to speak at all. Yet, as we see with Bill, there can be important reasons beneath the surface for why something needs saying again. And even if the person simply wants to 'hold the floor' for a while (be listened to with attention), it's a good idea to think twice before closing down conversations simply because they're a bit repetitive.

Danuta Lipinska is an experienced and expert therapist. Many of the techniques she's used with clients living with a dementia are standard for therapeutic work with everyone. That in itself is a lesson for us. You don't always have to treat people living with a dementia differently from how you'd treat anyone else. They deserve the same attention, respect and kindness that we'd give to others – and that's a topic we'll return to in Chapter 7.

But first, we need to explore two important topics that help us understand why Danuta's approach was so effective for Bill. In Chapter 4, we'll be asking: How does effective communication work? But before that, we address a more fundamental question: Why do we communicate? The answers to these two questions go to the heart of understanding why communication can get difficult when someone is living with a dementia.

---

4   Davis and Maclagan (2013, p. 102)
5   Guendouzi (2013, pp. 44–45)

Why do we communicate?

The ability to communicate – and to use language in particular – is universal across time, cultures and societies. Furthermore, children go through an extremely lengthy process of language acquisition to develop the necessary skills. It takes most infants a good year of observation and experimentation before they produce their first recognizable words, and another year to produce 50–100 words (though they understand a lot more), and put two words together into mini-'sentences' like *mummy shoe*. It's not till they're well past their third birthday that they make themselves understood in a similar way to adults. That's more than three years of attention and learning, full-time through their waking hours. It's a massive investment of effort.

The payoff for all that effort is that our communication tools – particularly language – allow us to achieve many important goals, including finding things out, being helpful, feeling important, avoiding getting lonely and influencing others. I'll argue in what follows that all of these goals, and more, are aspects of a single, vital drive – to *survive* (though I'll need to define 'survive' fairly broadly).

Communicating to survive

We're familiar with the idea that survival is the core driver in the natural world. Through natural selection, creatures evolve to maximize their chances of living long enough to reproduce. When they reproduce, they pass on the genes that carry the advantageous survival traits. Communication of one kind or another is very often central to this process. For example, flowers look and smell attractive to pollinators, and fruits are tasty to birds and animals so they get eaten and the seeds get dispersed. Animals develop spines, poisons, bright colours and disguises to warn off predators. Many creatures use displays of sound, colour and size to compete successfully for a mate. The most ancient ancestors of humans undoubtedly participated in this race for survival, using whatever methods of communication they had by then. Modern humans have language as an additional part of the package.

Language is very different from other kinds of communication. That's because the building blocks (sounds, words, and so on) represent meaning only indirectly. When a bird fluffs up its feathers against a rival, it's making itself look bigger in order to signal *look, I'm bigger than you thought*. There's something very direct about that – because bigger is bigger. Language, on the other hand, uses sounds that are in themselves meaningless, and combines them into words that are allotted meanings on, essentially, a random basis.[6] There's no point asking why English combines the sounds *k*, *a* and *t* to represent feline creatures, while Hindi combines *b*, *i*, *l* and *i*, and Swahili combines *p*, *a*, *k* and *a*. There's no way to predict what the word for 'cat' will be in a language you haven't come across before (unless it's historically related to a language you already know, which is how the German and French words for cat both turn out to be rather like the English one[7]).

Because languages are made up of abstract symbols, they have to be learnt through observation by each new generation – a very time-consuming process. The payoff comes from the massive range of meanings they can express. This range is possible because of the large number of individual words and the ways they can be combined into different structures. We can describe objects and actions, refer to relationships between ideas, talk about the past, present and future, speculate about events that have never happened and signal very subtle shades of meaning by choosing one word or phrase over another.

Is all this really necessary for our survival, though? It's hard to argue that we'd starve if we didn't have quite so many words for types of boat, or if we couldn't rephrase *The cat chased the bird* as *The bird was chased by the cat*. It all seems rather trivial, compared with having enough to eat and not getting killed by a leopard (which is what, we assume, kept our ancient ancestors on their toes). But it's not quite that simple.

---

6 Sign languages uses sequences of movements, and although some of them derive from imitative gestures (they are *iconic* rather than *symbolic*), there is still plenty of abstractness, such that sign languages need to be learnt. You can't just watch someone signing and automatically understand what they mean.

7 The German for cat is *Katze* and the French for cat is *chat*.

As the human brain got bigger, the human way of life became more complex. Language gave us additional ways to keep ourselves safe. It enables us to name and explain the difference between poisonous and edible plants, for example. Being able to tell other people things they wouldn't otherwise know means we can all learn indirectly from instruction, rather than having to discover everything for ourselves. There's no need for every child to discover that unripe fruit can give you stomach ache if adults can simply tell them not to eat it.

Having said all that, when we're dealing with socially and cognitively modern humans, it does make sense to broaden the meaning of 'survive'. Of course, it's still the case today that we must first attend to the absolute basics of air, water and food, or we'll die. But once we've got those secure, we humans start to build up many expectations, preferences and opportunities for enhancing our *quality* of life. We want to be interested, amused and challenged. We want to engage with others in activities we can't do on our own. And we want to build deep emotional bonds through the trust of sharing knowledge about each other. These are the experiences that help us feel fully alive, and when we don't have them, we can start to feel as if part of us is dying. In that sense, at least, they are necessary for our 'survival'.

Modifying our world

Creating our ideal world around us is our constant occupation. The world is a big and complicated place, and, annoyingly, it isn't organized around us or for our specific benefit. As a result, we frequently find a mismatch between how we'd like the world to be and how it actually is. When that happens, we must either put up with the discomfort of an unmet need or want, or intervene to make changes to our world that will benefit us.

When we can make changes for ourselves, no one else needs to be involved. For instance, if we're in danger, we'll get out of harm's way. If we're thirsty, we'll get ourselves something to drink if we can. If the room is too warm or cold, we can open or close the window.

But there are many, many things we'd like to change in our world that are beyond our direct reach, whether literally or metaphorically.

And then we need to get others to help us. If the products on the top shelf in the supermarket are too high for me, I'll need to get help from someone taller. If I want to see my doctor, I need to enlist the help of the receptionist in getting an appointment. If I go to a bar and want a beer, I need to get the bartender to pour it for me. If I want to know how my friend got on at her job interview, I need to ask her. And if she didn't get the job and I want her to know I feel sad for her, I need to tell her so. These are all examples of changes we might want to make to our world that have to involve someone else if they're to be brought about.

Most people recruit others to make changes to their world many, many times a day, whether face to face, by phone or using computer-mediated methods like email and social media. Even online shopping, automated as it is, ultimately connects the human who's responsible for making or supplying the item with the human who wants to own it. Communication is the way we convey to the other person what we want them to do. Whether it's shouting at someone to get out of our way or asking them nicely if they mind us eating the last strawberry, we use communication to get our message across.

But there's an obvious puzzle here. Why would *you* want to help me make *my* world better? What's in it for you? Why would you tolerate my being so self-centred?

Why do others support our agendas?

The first issue is whether my starting point here is even valid. I've just suggested that communication is self-serving. But don't we often put ourselves out for others, giving them information, explaining things, taking an interest in them, and so on, without any obvious benefit to ourselves? And surely there are many uses of communication that are relatively neutral. What's the 'survival' benefit of my messaging my friend to comment on the hairstyle of someone on TV, or chatting with a stranger on the bus about the state of the roads? I want to argue that even this sort of selfless or neutral activity is still driven, in the end, by the speaker's goal of getting their world to be as good as it can be. To see why, let's unwrap the issue a little.

For a start, it clearly doesn't make sense to suggest that speakers are selfish, while listeners just do whatever the speaker asks. If it were like that, no one would be keen on listening, and then speaking wouldn't be very effective. One way or another, we have to assume that listeners don't really mind responding in the way the speaker wants. So, there must be some benefits to that. What might they be?

Humans are cognitively and socially complex animals. So one explanation is that we often genuinely want things that will benefit others. Putting ourselves out for someone might temporarily inconvenience us yet give us the benefit of knowing we're making that sacrifice. Of course, if we actually *want* to put others first, it means we're using the speaker's needs to make a change that we want to our *own* world, which makes it all sound a bit self-serving again.[8]

Another possibility is that we're good at seeing the bigger picture – the balance of give and take. Listeners might be willing to tolerate being 'used' by speakers to an extent, because they know that in a minute it'll be their turn to be speaker and to 'use' the other person.

However, it could be even more complicated than that. Every time I say something to you, I upset the balance of your world slightly, leaving you wanting to do something to stabilize or change it. This, I believe, helps explain why listeners respond. Here's an example of how the balance of benefits shifts between the participants. Suppose I need to know the way to the railway station and I stop you on the street to ask you. My aim is to change my world from one in which I don't know which direction to go in, to one in which I do. Through what I say, I change your world. Before, it was one in which you were just going about your business. But I've turned it into one in which you've been asked a question and you haven't responded. Or, to put it another way, it's become a world in which a stranger is standing in front of you with an unmet need. Most people, faced with such a situation, would prefer to be in a world in which they've met that need, so that this unfinished business is tidied up and they can move on. In addition, you might realize that telling me where the station

---

8   For a discussion of whether it's ever possible to be completely selfless, see Wray (2020b, pp. 165–167).

is won't make your world any *worse*, whereas if you ignore me you might feel guilty later.

But you may want more. You might like the idea of my being very grateful that you were so neighbourly. To achieve this, you'll need to reply to me in a manner that encourages me to respond with gratitude. Perhaps you'll look at your watch impatiently, to signal that this really is quite inconvenient. In doing so, you change my world into one in which I feel a little guilty for bothering you. Once I get the subtle message that I should express gratitude, I'm likely to do so. It's a small reward that's easy to provide, since I genuinely am grateful.

We can see from that example that even a simple interaction is quite intricate. We are managing the needs and preferences of two people, not one, and that involves anticipating the likely behaviour of the other person in various possible scenarios. This 'mindreading' is very central to effective communication, and we'll look at it in more detail in Chapter 5.

When we don't get what we wanted

Before we explore further the process of getting others to help us make changes to our world, it's worth mentioning the limitations of that strategy. We obviously can't guarantee that others will always respond in the way we want. They might respond differently by mistake, if they draw the wrong conclusions about what we were aiming for, or if they misunderstand the situation. And sometimes, people just don't want to cooperate.

It's very often our understanding of the situation, and what we think it means for us, that decides how we respond when others communicate with us. And that helps explain why communication so easily goes awry when one of the participants is living with a dementia. It's not uncommon for two participants to have different perceptions of the situation, and that's a recipe for misunderstanding, disappointment and frustration. In the next chapter we'll look at the part played by the situation – or context – in making communication work.

ACTION POINTS FOR PEOPLE
LIVING WITH A DEMENTIA

1. Do you tend to repeat yourself? If you do, here are some strategies that might help you and others:

    a. Ask people to be understanding. Tell them that if you say something more than once, it's probably important in some way.

    b. Think about how you react to other people if they repeat themselves, and why you react like that. This may help you understand the reactions you get from others.

    c. If you do repeat yourself, would you prefer the other person to tell you so? Or should they respond as if they're hearing what you say for the first time? Why not talk to them about how it feels for you when they react in different ways.

2. Which aspects of your world are you most keen to change and protect these days? For instance:

    a. Which sorts of decisions do you especially want to make for yourself, and which are you happy for others to make for you?

    b. Which relationships are you most keen to protect, and which do you mind about less?

    c. Which of your hobbies and interests do you most want to continue with?

Keep this list handy so you can make these things your priority.

3. Think of someone you spend time with frequently. What do you imagine they most want to change and protect in their world? Understanding this might shed light on why they behave in certain ways and say the things they do.

4. It's important for all of us to feel useful and valued. You and the people close to you need to jointly find ways to feel useful and valuable to each other. Start that conversation by telling others how much you value them. Then you can say that, with their help, you'd like to find ways to do things for them too.

ACTION POINTS FOR FAMILIES, FRIENDS AND PROFESSIONALS

1. Think about which aspects of your world you're most keen to change and protect. Typical examples are: wanting to get things done without unnecessary difficulty; keeping in control emotionally; feeling useful and valued; not falling out with people. Now try and do the same for the person/people living with a dementia whom you care for or engage with. Understanding the sorts of things they most want to control in their world might help explain what they say and do.

2. Think of occasions when you tried to get someone to help you achieve something and it didn't work (e.g. you couldn't get the information you wanted; someone refused your request, or didn't understand it).

    a. How did you feel, and how did you react? What did you do to make yourself feel better about it? What could you or the other person have done to make the situation less difficult for you?

    b. People living with a dementia will often have feelings like the ones you've just recalled. What could you do to avoid making things worse for them? How could you help them feel better?

3. If a person living with a dementia whom you know tends to repeat themselves, how have you reacted? Which reactions work best? For instance, does it help to tell them that they've said/asked that before? If you end up having to answer the same question many times, what ways have you found for coping with your feelings about having to do so?

ACTION POINTS FOR BYSTANDERS

1. Think back to a situation when you interacted with a person living with a dementia.

    a. What do you think they were trying to achieve through what they said to you, and do you think they were successful?

   b. When you spoke, what were you trying to achieve, and were you successful?

   c. Can you think of ways to maximize how successful each of you is?

2. Sometimes, people who only have occasional contact with people living with a dementia find it easier to cope with communication challenges than those who are in the situation more often. Based on your own experiences so far:

   a. What advice would you give to others who occasionally engage with people living with a dementia or who have a full caring role about how to manage communication challenges?

   b. And what advice would you ask for from them?

CHAPTER FOUR

What Does Communication Involve?

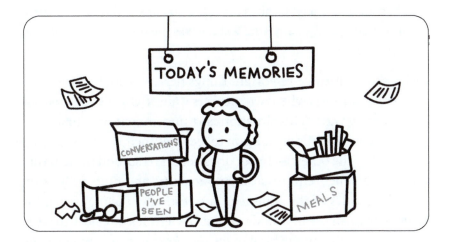

What I intended to communicate was...

One of the most moving and informative accounts of dementia I've read is *Alzheimer's from the Inside Out* by Richard Taylor.[1] It's people like him, dealing day by day with the direct experience of living with a dementia, who give us most insight into the impact of the disease. He writes openly about what he can and can't do, how he feels and how others treat him.

Taylor recounts telling his family that, when his present dog died, he'd like a new one. His family said it wasn't a good idea: you can't

---

1   Taylor (2007)

take care of a dog, we don't want the extra responsibility, dogs pee on the floor, leave hairs everywhere and can't be left alone. They said, 'Can't you understand why we don't want another dog?' and he replied, 'Can't you understand why I want another dog?' Reflecting on this conversation, he comments:

> What they *intended* to communicate was, 'we already feel inadequate and overwhelmed, taking care of you. Give us a break, and when there is an opportunity for us to have less responsibility, let us have it. Please. Especially if it only means not having a dog.' What I intended to communicate was, 'I am already feeling insecure and lonely. The thought of not having another dog giving me unconditional love when all that I need to do is provide two cups of food a day, some ear rubbing, and a daily long walk makes me even more frightened of the future.'[2]

Taylor shows us three important things here. The first is how disagreements can arise, when two speakers want to change their worlds in conflicting ways. This situation isn't uncommon of course. And it isn't uncommon for one person to feel that their wishes are being overruled by the other, as Taylor does here. The second thing is that resolving conflict requires at least one party, and preferably both, to see both sides of the argument. Interestingly, Taylor, despite his Alzheimer's, can see his family's point of view. It's not clear to what extent his family can see his, but let's assume they can, and just feel they can't meet his need for a replacement dog. This brings us to the third thing we learn from Taylor's account. Seeing a situation from both sides isn't itself a guarantee that a problem can be solved. Both Taylor and his family have needs and priorities and they just don't match up. However, when people can see each other's point of view, there's more likely to be understanding and negotiation, rather than an argument.

Elsewhere in his book, Taylor says that he would like caregivers to understand better how the world looks from his point of view: 'Most people offer answers to their own questions, not mine. My

---

2   Taylor (2007, p. 159)

questions, when answered by others, sound and feel to me as if people are avoiding my concerns and concentrating on their own "issues".[3] 'I just want others to try every day to figure me out, to understand me.'[4]

As we'll see in this chapter, understanding how the world looks to someone else isn't just about being more considerate. Unless we can add that information to our total picture of the *context* that we're operating in, we're likely to miss out on achieving our own goals.

Communication is a bit like table tennis. At first glance, it seems to be quite straightforward – I say something, you say something back, I say something back, and so on, till one of us smashes the point and wins. But neither table tennis nor communication is actually that simple. Table tennis isn't just about hitting a ball back and forth. It's not even just about the rules for scoring points. It's about how the players understand the dynamics of the ball's flight: when exactly the ball will make contact with the bat, how hard to hit the ball to get it to travel the desired distance, what precise hand movement will send the ball at a specific angle or spin it. And it's about how players interpret the opponent's moves: where they're most likely to direct the ball to, what happens to the ball if the opponent steps forwards or backwards while hitting it, how the opponent will return a drop shot or a smash. Considerations of at least as much complexity underpin the moment-by-moment choices and judgements of a successful communicator.

In the next sections, we'll look at how communication works from the point of view of first the speaker and then the listener. For simplicity, I'm focusing on spoken communication. Of course, writing and sign language are also options, and what I say next can be fairly easily adapted to cover them.

---

3   Taylor (2007, p. 31)
4   Taylor (2007, p. 218)

The communication procedure for the speaker

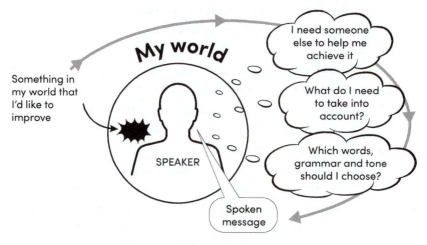

Figure 4.1: The speaker's procedure

What does communicating involve then? Figure 4.1 illustrates the process. As we saw in Chapter 3, the first step is noticing that something isn't quite perfect for us – represented in the diagram by the black explosion within 'My world'. This is what we want to change. For instance, we might want some physical improvement, such as making the room warmer, or getting a cold drink, or making sure the grass is cut. We might want a world in which we know something we currently don't know, such as how to make lasagne or whether a delivery has arrived yet. We might want a world in which we've provided information to someone else. Or we might want to feel reassured, comforted or challenged. Those are just a few examples. We live complicated lives, and we're trying to make little changes to our world all the time.

Once we know what we want to change, we need to work out how to change it. Sometimes, we can, of course, change things without anyone's help – switch on the heating, go to the fridge for a drink, and so on. But we'll just focus here on when we can't make the change for ourselves, and we need to get someone else to do something for us, as indicated in the top thought bubble. Now we have to work out how to make that happen: what we need to take into account, and how we should formulate what we say, as in the middle and lower thought bubbles.

For example, imagine I hear that my friend Charles is having a party that I haven't been invited to. I'd really like to go, and that means I need to get an invitation – this is the change I want to make to my world. I can't just invite myself. I need to persuade Charles to invite me. What do I need to take into account, to achieve this? First, I need to consider my options. I could phone Charles directly, and if I do, I could ask him straight out if I can come. Or I could pretend I called for a different reason and then try to move things to a point where he admits he's having the party and invites me. Alternatively, I could contact my friend Melanie, who's already invited, and get her to ask Charles if I can come.

Which choice I make will depend on what I know about Charles, Melanie and the situation – all this information that I need to take into account is the *context*. Here are some potential considerations when trying to get my party invitation. Melanie's really talkative. If I try to get the invitation by calling her, she might stay on the phone for ages, with knock-on effects for the rest of my day. If I contact Charles and ask him directly if I can come, he might say *no*, or say *yes* but hesitantly and then I'll feel hurt. It might also put him in an awkward position, with consequences for next time we meet. If I phone Charles and hope he invites me without my asking, how will I feel if I'm unsuccessful?

Let's say I choose the option of phoning Charles but not asking directly for an invitation. Now I have to work out what to say, and how, so things go in the direction I want. I decide to start off by being very friendly and asking him about himself, so he's reminded of what a nice person I am (the perfect party guest). I'll then ask him if he's seen Melanie recently. I hope he'll say she's coming to his party and invite me too. If that doesn't work, I'll ask him if he's got a busy weekend planned. If he doesn't mention the party, I'll know he definitely doesn't want to invite me, and I can close the conversation before anyone gets embarrassed.

This may sound extremely calculating and even devious, but when we communicate, we generally do make many such careful judgements and decisions, to shape what we say and how we say it. Only like that can we steer towards getting the change to our world that we want without any unintended changes along the way.

All of this shows how we draw on various bits of knowledge, assumptions and beliefs to reach our goal successfully. They are part, but not all, of the context information we use. Other parts of the context include what happened last time we were in this situation, what we know about the listener's personality and circumstances, and so on. So my approach to Charles could be shaped by, say, whether I've been invited to his parties in the past, whether I've ever accepted an invitation and not turned up, whether he and I had an argument recently, whether I think he can afford to invite more people, whether he's shy or outgoing, how at ease I feel when talking to him, and so on. Furthermore, I'll use context to decide the best time to phone him, and even which language to use when I speak to him, if we both know more than one.

Returning to Figure 4.1, once we've assessed the context, we can decide which words, grammar and tone of voice to use for conveying our message. We also choose non-verbal gestures, facial expressions, and so on at this stage. In assembling the message, we're shaping not only *what* we say, but how it comes across – as breathless, strident, humorous, friendly or whatever.

Finally, we activate the mechanical processes for turning the planned utterance into speech. This involves lining up a lot of physical movements in the vocal apparatus – from lungs to lips – so that the sounds come out accurately and in the right order. The sounds travel across the air and are picked up by the ears of the listener.

The communication procedure for the listener

Figure 4.2 shows what happens when the listener receives the package of sounds. The process begins in the bottom right when the sounds are identified as a message. It's not a foregone conclusion that sense can be made of these sounds. For instance, if the speaker mistakenly chooses a language the listener doesn't understand, then the communication will break down at that point. But assuming the listener does know the language the speaker used, then, as Figure 4.2 shows, the next job is identifying the words, grammar and tone that have been used. This information gives the listener the *surface* or literal level of the meaning. For instance, suppose I say to Charles, *I'm not doing anything on Saturday* in a rather sad voice, then at this stage in the process, Charles simply understands a statement of a fact and that I sounded sad when I said it.

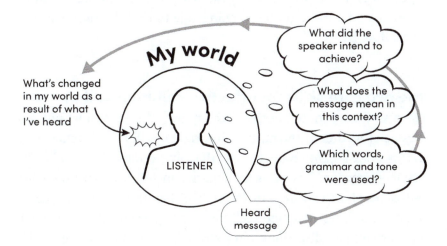

What did the speaker intend to achieve?

What's changed in my world as a result of what I've heard

My world

LISTENER

What does the message mean in this context?

Which words, grammar and tone were used?

Heard message

Figure 4.2: The listener's procedure

It's at the next two levels up that Charles will look for the deeper meaning in what I said – what my comment signifies in the context as he sees it. He'll think (I hope), *Why has she told me that? Ah, perhaps she'd like to come to the party herself.* I've fed him a piece of apparently neutral information, which adds to his context knowledge. He can now re-evaluate everything he knows and come up with a thought he hadn't had before – to invite me to the party. I never actually told him I wanted to come to the party, and yet somehow I got him to do what I wanted.

We can see how crucial the listener's role is in whether speakers get the changes they want to their world. Nothing's going to change unless the listener responds in the desired way. It's up to the speaker to pick just the right way of expressing the message. Speakers can't *make* listeners act. All they can do is try to control how the listener relates the message to the context. They can't know exactly how the context looks to the listener, though they can certainly develop skills for guessing. The speaker's success, then, relies on seeing the context from the other person's point of view as well as their own, so they accurately anticipate how a message will come across.

For the rest of this chapter, we're going to look in even more detail at how context works, because we'll see in Chapter 5 that when a person is living with a dementia, it's context that creates most problems – far more than not being able to find the right word or speak fluently.

The two core skills for effective communication

As we've just seen, to get the outcome we want, we must put our message together in the most appropriate way for the listener. This means assessing the context. To do that, we need two core skills. The first is *observation*. Observing the situation includes working out what the listener is in a position to do. A wheelchair user can't be expected to get something off a high shelf for us, and we wouldn't usually ask a young child for directions in the street. The second skill we need is *mindreading*. We need to work out how our message will come across to the other person, by assessing what they already know, what they're expecting, and what they'll consider appropriate and acceptable.

Let's first consider the matter of what they already know. Figure 4.3 shows the relationship between our knowledge and someone else's. Mindreading involves assessing what the other person knows, and which parts of what they know they believe we also know or don't know. Suppose I walk into an ice cream parlour and say, *One double chocolate and one single caramel with toffee, please*. My choice of words has been made on the basis of many judgements about what the assistant already knows, including these: we're in an ice cream parlour; it's your job to serve me; when I say *one double chocolate* I'm referring to a large helping of a type of ice cream you serve; when I refer to *toffee* I'm referring to a type of sauce you serve; I'm expecting the ice creams to be supplied in two separate suitable receptacles for holding and carrying. None of this information is directly stated, yet I can make myself understood because of my accurate assumptions about what the assistant knows and, importantly, what he believes *I* know and assume (e.g. he assumes that I trust he will actually serve me ice cream and not some poisonous look-alike).

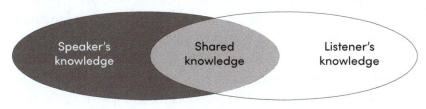

Figure 4.3: Separate and shared knowledge

My mindreading also helps me understand what he's expecting. He's expecting that I've come into the parlour to buy ice cream, not to sell him insurance, so I don't need to explain what I want. He's also expecting that I know what ice cream is and what it tastes like. So, he won't be warning me that it's cold and sweet. On the other hand, he might *not* be sure I'll know it could contain traces of nuts. So, I anticipate he might check that the risk of nuts is in our shared knowledge space, not just in his knowledge space, while being absent from mine. Finally, he's expecting that I'll pay for the ice creams and carry them away from the counter, so he can serve the next person. I need to know that he expects these things, otherwise I won't understand what he's trying to achieve when he tells me the cost and, after I've paid, says *goodbye*.

Managing listeners' expectations

Each person we communicate with is different. Each person has a background and a set of expectations built on their previous experience, preferences, fears, enthusiasms, and so on. Our relationship with each person is unique too. With people we already know, memory helps us build up a map of the roles we play relative to each other, what's happened between us in the past, and what information we both know. As we'll see later, the role of memory is central in understanding what goes wrong in communication when someone's living with a dementia.

With people we haven't met before, our observational and mind-reading skills guide our judgements about how to approach them. We look for clues in their dress, behaviour, posture and speech patterns to guess how polite they'll expect us to be, and which language, dialect or accent they'll expect us to use. We evaluate what they're likely to know, and what words will be most appropriate for them. For instance, when we talk to children, we typically use simpler vocabulary; the same can apply for some people living with a dementia. Some words have different meanings or connotations for people of different generations. For example, someone who doesn't use the internet might be confused by references to *the cloud* or to *following* someone. Some older people recall when *wireless* referred to a radio set and a *troll* was an ugly creature who terrorized a family of goats crossing a bridge.

When I wrote the first draft of Chapter 2 of this book in February 2020, I wanted to describe what happens when someone gets a dementia diagnosis and then finds that their friends and neighbours withdraw from them. I chose to express this idea as 'social distancing', which was not a phrase I particularly knew, but one that seemed to capture the idea well. By the time I was redrafting the chapter in April 2020, the term 'social distancing' had a completely new meaning because of the Covid-19 pandemic. I had to find a new way to express my idea, because I anticipated that readers would now think of a quite different concept from the one I meant.

Keeping up

When we're interacting with others, we're never in quite the same place twice. Each time we say or do something, we change our own world and the world of the other person. Whatever we said last time, and however we said it, might have worked then, but that doesn't guarantee it'll work now. Each time we judge how to use communication to get others to change our world for us, we have to look at the situation on its own merits.

For instance, imagine a mother has just made dinner and wants her son to come and eat. She says, *It's dinner time*. Note, by the way, that *It's dinner time* isn't actually an instruction, invitation or request in itself, just an observation. It's an established statement that's usually enough to get people to come to the table, because they use their mindreading skills to recognize why it's been said.

So far so good. But five minutes later, the lad still hasn't turned up. So, the mother goes back to him. The world isn't the same as last time, because she's already told him about dinner once. So, she probably won't just say *It's dinner time* in exactly the same way. She might begin *I said...* and use a louder voice or more marked intonation. This signals to him that *she* knows she's told him already and also that she knows *he* knows it. As we'll see in Chapter 6, it's not uncommon for people living with a dementia not to recall that you said something before. As a result, they could be very confused or disconcerted when they get the *second-time* presentation instead of the more neutral first-time one they were expecting.

Three or more people in the conversation

So far, we've only considered conversations involving two people. Having more people makes the context more complicated, because, unless someone is ignored or regarded as unimportant, the context has to be separately evaluated for each person.

Let's imagine Jake is trying to persuade Eliza to lend him some money so he can go out for a beer. However, Harriet is also present. Although he's only directly addressing Eliza, he's got to work out how Harriet might react to what she hears. He borrowed money off Harriet last week and never repaid it. If Harriet hadn't been there, he'd have promised Eliza to pay her back tomorrow. But he can't do that now, because there's a risk that his world will change for the worse. For instance, Harriet might tell Eliza not to believe his promise. Or she might get angry about Eliza getting repaid before she does.

Suppose he's now asked Eliza for the money. Eliza doesn't trust him to pay it back. The world she wants is one in which she doesn't lend him money. However, she doesn't want to hurt his feelings. If Harriet weren't present, she'd just tell Jake that she's broke. But

Harriet saw her with a handful of notes an hour ago. She doesn't want to create a world in which Harriet knows she's a liar and thinks she's mean.

So, the more people present, the more complicated the calculations about the context. We'll explore more deeply in Chapter 5 why it can be so difficult for people living with a dementia to keep up, when more than one other person is in the conversation. But there's one situation worth considering here. Let's suppose Beryl and her husband Colin are at the memory clinic, because Beryl is having some difficulties that might be signs of dementia. Colin very much wants to hear from the specialist what the diagnosis is, and what to expect in the future. But because Beryl is in the room, he's reluctant to ask, in case the information upsets or frightens her. He has a conflict between two different things he wants, each associated with a different person. Success with one outcome puts the other at risk.

One option he considers is getting a chat with the specialist on his own. However, Colin feels that talking about Beryl behind her back would be disloyal and disrespectful, something that would make him feel guilty, changing his world for the worse. Colin decides to ask the specialist if there's any written information relevant to their situation. In this way, he hopes to collect what he needs in pamphlets and information sheets, while shielding Beryl from the content. However, for this to work, it's vital that the specialist understands why he's chosen this approach and doesn't, for example, hand copies to both of them and start talking through the content. We shouldn't be surprised if Colin can't find a way to successfully manage this situation, stressed as he already is. He may leave the meeting without having got the information he needs.

The role of memory, information management and concentration in communication

At first glance, the two core skills of effective communication – observation and mindreading – might appear to be independent of memory. But they're not. How can you to interpret what you observe unless you know what *else* has happened and can swiftly merge old and new information? How can you guess what the other person is thinking, unless you can recall what they've just said and done, who they are and why you're having the conversation?[5]

Memory, concentration and the ability to manage information efficiently are often casualties in dementia, as we saw in Chapter 1. Many people's dementia is directly associated with an impairment to short-term and/or long-term memory. But even people without memory impairments can find they don't recall certain information. This could be because events happened too fast for them to take everything in, or because they got distracted and so didn't notice what was going on or what was said.

The brain damage associated with dementia-causing diseases tends to reduce the speed and efficiency of information processing. The processing burden on someone living with a dementia could be at least as heavy as it is for someone without dementia who's tired, unwell and a little drunk, as they attempt to do several difficult tasks at once, with a lot of background distractions. It's a lot to cope with.

Human memory is complicated, and so is its role in creating difficulties with communication when someone's living with a dementia. We don't need to dig into all the detail here,[6] but there are some particularly important observations that will set the scene for later chapters. The take-home message is that someone with memory problems is going to struggle to assess all the context. And if they can't do that, they're in a weak position to put messages together in the most appropriate way for getting the outcome they want.

The importance of episodic memory

Our *episodic* memory is our memory for events. It's one of the types of so-called *explicit* memory – where we know we know something and we can say what it is we know.[7] For instance, I recall feeding the cat this morning, and I can talk about knowing it and how I know:

---

5 See Guendouzi (2013) for the importance of such information to people living with a dementia.

6 For a detailed exploration of memory in the dementia communication context, see Wray (2020b, chapter 3).

7 For a helpful overview of the nature of episodic memory, see Tulving (2002).

I remember, because there was an item on the radio about cat food just as I spooned the food into the dish, and I thought what a coincidence that was. The other type of explicit memory is our knowledge of facts – *semantic* memory. This encompasses things like knowing what the capital of France is, the names of flowers in the garden and why vegetables are better for us than deep-fried pizza. Often, semantic and episodic memory work together. Semantic memory tells you where you went to school, which is a fact that you could know even without recalling going there; and episodic memory takes you back to particular incidents so you can, in a sense, relive them.

In dementia, this close relationship between episodic and semantic memory sometimes gets disrupted. Suppose there's shouting in the street and it reminds someone of frightening events they witnessed as a child. Their long-term episodic memory might take them back to that time, so they re-experience the fear. This much can happen to anyone. However, people who aren't living with a dementia can immediately use their semantic memory to remind themselves that those events happened many years ago and are no longer a threat. They'll also use their episodic memory of events earlier in the day to reassure themselves they're not in that long-ago place now. Dementia can make it more difficult to bring these different streams of information together. When that happens, the strongest emotional reaction – in this case fear – quite naturally gets most prominence. Once someone's overwhelmed by strong emotions it's difficult for them to use other information to calm the feelings down.

Not all memory is explicit. We also have *implicit* memory, and one type is our knowledge of how to do things. We can learn very complicated series of actions and perform them perfectly without really having any conscious awareness of how we do them. A pianist may be able to play a piece beautifully but struggle to find effective words to explain how they get that effect. In dementia, implicit memory is generally not affected until very late on, if at all. In contrast, explicit episodic memory is often impaired at an early stage.

It's difficult to know for sure whether events get stored in episodic memory and then can't be reached, or whether in some types of dementia they simply never get laid down in memory at all. The net effect is the same – we're all familiar with situations in which, say, a person living with a dementia is asked if they enjoyed the outing they just went on, and they can't recall where they went, what they did or, perhaps, even that they went out at all.

This difficulty with episodic memory is well recognized and is a primary feature of Alzheimer's disease in particular. But the full impact of episodic memory impairment is much greater than just gaps in the person's knowledge about what's happened recently. That's because episodic memory has an important characteristic that's central to our sense of what we know and who we are.

Episodic memory and our sense of authority

Many of us have had the experience of disagreeing with a family member or friend about the details of some event in the past. Although both of us were there, we seem to remember the details differently. The reason we get so insistent that we're right and the other person's wrong is because we have a particular sense of authority about events we were present at. We feel deeply in our bones that our recall is correct *because we were there*.[8]

We have much more confidence in our episodic memories than we do in our semantic memories. Everyone's semantic knowledge has equal status. If I claim that the bird that lays the largest egg is the swan, and you claim it's the ostrich, then your claim may well make me think, *Oh, perhaps I've remembered that fact wrong.* I won't feel the same sort of indignation as I would if you said, *No, when we saw the Queen, her hat was pink, not yellow.*

But how could it come about that two people at the same event remember it differently? Whenever we recall events from our past, we relive them in a way. In our mind's eye, we're back there, experiencing them again. But this can cause problems because we're obviously not

---

8   This strong sense of self within our episodic memories is referred to by Tulving (2002) as 'autonoetic awareness'.

really back there. Rather, we're reimagining the events.[9] Over time, we can introduce thoughts and interpretations that weren't part of the original event. Then, having imagined them into the scene, they become part of the memory. In other words, the more times we recall an event, the more it's likely to get changed. We might blend two events into one or introduce details that make logical sense (such as 'remembering' that the Queen was wearing a yellow hat, because she often does).

So, there are two features of episodic memory that can come into conflict. On the one hand, because we were there, we feel a strong sense of authority about being right in what we recall. On the other hand, what we recall might have got changed over the years. That's how someone else can be just as certain as I am about what colour the Queen's hat was on the day of the visit, but have a different colour in mind. Both of us have that deep sense of knowing we're right. If we discover in the records that in fact her hat was blue, we're both likely to claim with a great deal of confidence that the official record is wrong. We should know, after all, because we were there!

It's very important to us emotionally to assert our right to knowledge about our own experiences because we feel we *own* them. But when people are living with a dementia, several things happen that put that self-confidence in jeopardy. One is that they find gaps where some of those memories should be. Someone tells them they were present at an event, but they can't recall that they were. Someone insists they were told a particular piece of information five minutes ago, but they have no memory of it. This is alarming, because it's as if they're disappearing – they weren't present in their own life experiences.

A second difficulty is that when others pick up on the fact that someone's having memory difficulties, they immediately assume that the person's always going to be the one who's mistaken. Like hyenas, they home in on the weakness in order to feed their own sense of authority. All those arguments that previously were fairly evenly matched (*I'm certain the Queen had a yellow hat – No, I'm certain*

---

9   This idea, much written about in current psychology, dates back at least as far as the 17th-century writings of the philosopher John Locke (1690, X:2).

it was pink) start to be weighted against the person living with the dementia. If the other person has remembered an event differently (they, of course, may also have reinvented the facts), they're going to argue that they're right and they'll probably win. The person living with the dementia may feel very deeply that actually their own recollection is more accurate (and they may be right) but they will also start to doubt their own judgement, because they know they have memory difficulties.

Overall, these experiences will whittle away at a person's self-belief. Richard Taylor makes the following important observation:

> I have now started to check with people to make sure that I know the difference between my own recollections (which I want to believe are always true) and the recollections of others... sometimes I am correct in my recollections and others are the ones who are confused and do not immediately know it. I still know this to be true, at least once in a while. Others who know I have Alzheimer's generally assume that they are correct and that my disease causes me to be incorrect. When my recollections are corrected based on the generalization that my disease guarantees I am wrong, I lose another ounce of self-confidence in my ability to know and remember what is going on around me.[10]

Episodic memory and identity

It's often been pointed out that in the modern industrialized world, people are not so much human *beings* as human *doings*. In other words, we create our sense of identity less from our inherent personality traits, our feelings and our moment-by-moment experience of the world in the present, than from the things we've done, the places we've been, the money we've made, the people we've met and the evidence we've accumulated that we are, in the eyes of others, *someone*. Clocking up our identity in this way is very dependent on being able to recall all that information. As people's dementia progresses, they can struggle to bring the details of their life back

---

10 Taylor (2007, p. 154)

to mind. Without memories of key events, a person's life story and, hence, identity, is depleted. It shouldn't surprise us, then, that people living with a dementia often say things like *I don't know who I am*.[11]

Memory impairment can affect identity in other ways as well. Perhaps someone used to be the expert on cricket trivia. But now they can't access that expertise – which is part of explicit semantic memory – and so can't claim that aspect of their identity. They're not the go-to person for that information, and they feel less useful and valued as a result.

Even deeper questions about memory and identity can arise. Some people wonder, *Who will I be when I have forgotten who I am?* and *Will my loved ones abandon me if they feel that the core 'me' is no longer there, particularly if I no longer know who they are?* People of faith might also ask, *How can I claim to love God if I have forgotten who God is?*[12]

The dread accompanying these deep anxieties is surely one of the reasons why dementia is feared so much. Sincere reassurances from family, friends and professionals may be of only limited help. But you may have come across the following inspirational anecdote: A man whose wife was living with a dementia visited her with faithful regularity. A friend said to him, 'Why do you continue to visit her, when she no longer knows who you are?' He replied, 'Because I still know who she is.'

Still knowing who someone is may rely more on our knowledge and memory of how the person used to be than on what can be observed now. But glimpses of their personality, including mysterious moments of lucidity when the person seems to have temporary access to lost faculties,[13] suggest that perhaps dementia is more a process of covering up the person's core being than totally destroying it.

Assisting people living with a dementia to reconnect with their own life stories has been the focus of David Clegg's work.[14] While employed as a care assistant in a residential care home, Clegg started

11   Clegg (2010, p. xviii)
12   Swinton (2012, pp. 3–4, 10)
13   For a short discussion of temporary lucidity, see Wray (2020b, p. 28).
14   Brown and Clegg (2007); Clegg (2010, 2015)

getting residents to tell him the stories of their lives. Even though care home managers told him that people with severe dementia could not be reached, he repeatedly uncovered fascinating information about them, simply by taking the trouble to ask. By talking with individuals over several months, Clegg built up written accounts of who they were and what they'd done in their life. As their dementia became worse, this information could be used to reignite memories they now struggled to retrieve. One of his participants commented, when Clegg was able to remind her of details she could no longer bring to mind, 'Oh... aren't you good! What a good memory... I was trying very hard to hang onto it.'[15]

Memory and communication

And now, as we combine these features of episodic memory with the earlier discussion in this chapter, comes the final twist of the knife. As episodic memories become more difficult to retrieve, people living with a dementia find it harder to draw together all the contextual information needed for effectively communicating with others. They're no longer sure what's just happened, and what the assumptions and beliefs of others currently are. They can't gauge what it's possible and reasonable to try to change in their world, or how to approach getting others to help. They're nervous of getting it wrong and annoying or upsetting someone, embarrassing themselves, and failing to make the change that they wanted.

The downward spiral starts with the unreliability of their memory, but, importantly, that's not why it progresses. The decline is driven by how other people respond to the memory difficulties of people living with a dementia. In particular, it's caused in large measure by the natural desire that other people have to be right and to preserve and protect their own authority and identity. They have their own need to keep a sense of authority about events they were part of. And that sets up battles that it's difficult for those living with a dementia to win.[16]

---

15   Clegg (2015, Shirley Session 13)
16   Wray (2020b, p. 52)

It's up to those without the memory impairment to recognize how easily they can undermine the confidence of people living with a dementia by reducing their capacity to have some control over their world. In the terms explored in Chapter 2, we who are not living with a dementia must take steps to build up and sustain the emotional reserve of those who are, so they're as resilient as possible against the unavoidable frustrations and disappointments caused by their compromised cognitive abilities. And when we do this as a society, we build up their social reserve too, because we create new ways for everyone to think about who people living with a dementia really are. In turn, that will help them stay in touch with the information that anchors their sense of identity.

ACTION POINTS FOR PEOPLE LIVING WITH A DEMENTIA

1. Think about an occasion when you tried to make a change in your world and weren't successful. What went wrong? What could you do next time to improve the chances of success?

2. When others speak to you, use the context to 'read between the lines'. What do they really want you to help them change in their world? For example, do they want some information from you? Do they want reassurance that you're okay? Do they need you to do something for them? This may help you decide how to respond most appropriately.

3. How do you feel when someone doesn't understand what you were trying to say, or if you don't understand them? Other people won't automatically realize how you feel. They may need your guidance about how to help. Try saying, *When that happened, I felt...* and *If that happens in the future, it'd be very helpful if you would...*

4. If you're concerned about your memory getting worse over time, could you write down a few of the happy memories and the pieces of information that you most want to hang on to. Link them to objects, smells or sounds (including music) that

will help you bring the details to mind in the future. By sharing this information with someone who cares about you, it should be possible to recall these memories longer.

ACTION POINTS FOR FAMILIES, FRIENDS AND PROFESSIONALS

1. Which sorts of changes that you try to make each day are least successful? To what extent might the failures be because you and the person living with the dementia have different understandings of the context – for example, what's important, what's possible, what the alternatives are, why it's relevant? Does realizing this give you any new options?
2. Practise asking yourself what the person living with the dementia might be trying to achieve when they say something. Remember to take into account goals hiding beneath the surface, such as getting reassurance. How could this understanding alter your response to them?
3. Cast your mind back to some occasion where you were certain that something had taken place as you recalled it, but someone else argued that you were wrong. How did you feel? Can this experience help you support people living with a dementia when it happens to them?

ACTION POINTS FOR BYSTANDERS

1. When you engage in conversations with people (whether living with a dementia or not), notice the assumptions that you each make for the communication to work effectively. How do you and they work out that information – for instance, by using location, appearance, past experience? If a person living with a dementia seems to have made assumptions that you haven't made, try guessing what the assumptions are to help you understand how they see the situation.

2. If a person living with a dementia doesn't seem to have un-derstood what you meant, think about which aspects of the situation they may not be sure of. Find ways to gently provide that information, such as reminding them of what you said earlier or explaining what you're doing.

CHAPTER FIVE

When Communication Goes Wrong

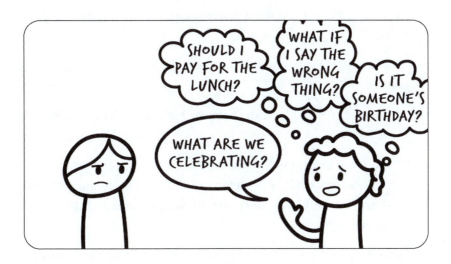

Val and her dad

Val Ormrod's father had been diagnosed with Alzheimer's. Val brought him to live with her and her husband, so she could support him more effectively. In her book *In My Father's Memory*,[1] she writes movingly about the experience – its challenges but also its many rewards. One morning, when she was helping him get up, the following conversation, directly quoted from her book, took place.

'I haven't got any sausages.'

---

1   Ormrod (2019)

He picks up his teeth from the bedside table, then his comb, then his eye drops. It's a familiar ritual in which he becomes agitated about something he can't find.

'I can't find anything. All my things have gone. Somebody's taken them.'

'Are they in the bathroom?'

'Someone takes them from there. When there's someone down there they take them.'

[...]

'Okay, so what do you want your sausages for?' I ask, trying to get a clue.

'You know.' He puts a hand up to his neck and makes a shaving gesture.

'Ah,' I say, fetching his razor from the bathroom. 'This is what you need.'

'I haven't got anything that you listen to,' he says, handing the razor back. He knows what he wants to say and most of the time he finds an alternative way of saying it. It's an electric razor and the battery has gone flat.[2]

In this extract we see Val figuring out her dad's meaning from the context (including his gestures) when he can't find the words he needs. When either of them speaks or gestures, the processes for planning and preparing a message take place (see Chapter 4, Figure 4.1). And when the other person hears or sees a message, the processes for unpacking take place (see Figure 4.2). We're going to look in detail at the start of the conversation, to see those processes in action. What should strike you is just how much ability Dad has in managing the communication processes.

---

2   Ormrod (2019, pp. 242–243)

Dad says 'I haven't got any sausages'

Dad has identified something in his world that he'd like to change – he'd like to find his razor. He needs to enlist Val's help to locate it. To do that, he's got to decide what to say to Val, to get her to respond in the way he wants. That means evaluating the context. We can't see inside his mind, it's true, but there are some important clues. First, he recognizes that Val is worth asking for help with this problem. Of course, he may not have much choice if she's the only person available, but he didn't ask the cat or the wardrobe. Despite his quite advanced Alzheimer's, he knows who can and can't help him. Second, he knows he can ask for help by using a descriptive statement rather than a request. He knows, in other words, that Val will understand *I haven't got any...* as meaning *please can you help me find...* This is a standard feature of communication, and he hasn't lost his ability to use it.

As he looks in his mental dictionary for the words he needs, Dad encounters a problem. He can't retrieve a key word he needs, *razor*. Of all the words to lose, this is the most inconvenient. But it isn't an uncommon problem. Don't we all end up saying *where's the what-dyamacallit* from time to time? It's the names for the very things we're focused on that most often escape us. On the other hand, notice all the language components he does come up with successfully. He creates a coherent sentence frame,[3] *I haven't got...* which indicates to Val what the problem is. The only thing she doesn't know is what it is he hasn't got.

It's interesting that he uses a plural noun, *sausages*, in place of the singular noun *razor*. Yet the sentence frame he's chosen is the grammatical one for the replacement, rather than the original. So, he says *any sausages*, where he presumably would have said *my, a* or *the razor*. This shows that his grammatical processing is working well.

---

3   A sentence frame is a grammatical sentence with one or more words missing. Frames are a convenient way to create an entire sentence without much effort. They can be tailor-made for the occasion by choosing the appropriate word(s) to slot in (for more on this topic, see Wray 2002). Consider how the song *Happy Birthday* works. The entire song is a frame with a gap for the name of the person whose birthday it is. The song itself is useful over and over again, yet because of that one modification each time, we also make it personal to the one individual it's intended for on that occasion.

Having put his sentence together internally, Dad is able to produce it fluently and comprehensibly, and the sounds carry through the air to Val.

Val interprets 'I haven't got any sausages'

Val receives the sounds and her brain recognizes, categorizes and unpacks them to identify the component words of Dad's utterance. She looks up the words in her mental dictionary and uses her grammatical knowledge to see how they relate to each other. This gives her the literal message *I haven't got any sausages*. Now, her job is to use context to make sense of what she's heard.

She recognizes that his statement has a purpose. He wants to change something in his world with her help. So, although it is, on the surface, a simple comment, she receives and interprets it as a request for her to help him find the 'sausages'. She's aided in this interpretation by the fact that he behaves in his customary agitated way, picking things up.

Now, she has to decide whether it literally is sausages that he wants. It's morning, and she's helping him get up, so presumably he's not had breakfast yet. Perhaps, then, he's simply saying what he'd like to eat. Why doesn't she interpret his statement that way? The reason is that she brings other bits of context into the mix. He's still in the process of getting up, and perhaps she considers it unlikely that he'd mention breakfast yet. Perhaps she knows he'd never request sausages for breakfast. But, most importantly, as Val has explained earlier in the book, her dad often uses *sausages* as a substitute for a word he can't find. So, she's alert to the likelihood that it's standing in for something else.

What happens in the rest of the conversation

Before Val can reply to Dad's comment about not having any sausages, he adds some more information: 'I can't find anything. All my things have gone. Somebody's taken them.' Why does he say this? We can't know, but it might be because he's uneasy with the state of his world. He's anxious that his first statement won't be enough to convince Val to help him. Again, we can see how much linguistic ability and contextual knowledge he's able to draw on. His new comment follows on from the previous one seamlessly, still using *them* to refer to a plural entity (the 'sausages'). He also uses a common strategy for getting attention – exaggeration. Even though he's actually touching some of his possessions as he speaks, he says that all his things have gone, just like a teenager might complain, *No one ever listens to me!* or an exasperated customer might say, *Nothing I've bought from here has ever been any good!*

On hearing his rather extreme claim, Val could have responded, *Don't be silly, there are plenty of your things here.* But she doesn't. That's because she uses context to help her evaluate what Dad really means to achieve. His statement isn't an accusation or complaint but an expression of loss of control. He doesn't need correcting or telling off but comforting and supporting. So, instead, she focuses on how she can best help him.

Her world is one in which her dad has asked her for help, but she's not sure what she has to do. She needs to change her world into one where she knows what *sausages* refers to. She also needs to signal to Dad that she's trying to help him. How can she achieve both? She could ask him directly, *What do you mean by 'sausages'?* But her knowledge of the context tells her that this isn't likely to achieve her goal of getting information, because he clearly can't find the word he needs. Furthermore, that question might come across as badgering him or criticizing him for making a mistake, which would undermine her second goal. So, she puts together a message that asks him if the 'sausages' are in the bathroom, judging that he may know the answer.

Dad's response, 'Someone takes them from there. When there's someone down there they take them,' might seem to indicate that he hasn't taken any notice of Val's question, but this can't be so. He clearly has received and unpacked the words, because in his reply he uses *there* to refer to the bathroom. So, why doesn't he answer her question? It might be because he doesn't know the answer. But he might be taking the answer for granted and moving straight to the next idea, by telling Val that, irrespective of whether the 'sausages' are usually there, they won't be there now. Jumping over part of the content, leaving the other person to work out the missing information, is something we all very commonly do. If I arrive at a bus stop and ask someone waiting there *Have you seen a number 57 go by?* the person might reply *They're always unreliable*. I will figure out from this reply that the answer to my question is *no*, even though it's not been said.[4] So, Dad isn't doing anything unusual by not replying directly.

Val's attempt to work out what 'sausages' are hasn't worked, so her world continues to be one in which she needs to help her dad but doesn't have enough information. She chooses another approach, asking him what they're used for. Again, we can see that Dad understands what she says and why she's saying it, because he gives a suitable response that can help her modify her world towards having the information she needs. Although he can't produce the language for his message, he uses mime very effectively.

Once Val gives him the razor, she assumes she's made his world okay. But she's wrong, because he can't use it till it's charged. Dad identifies in his own mind what needs to be changed in his world and again turns to Val as the person who can make that change happen. Again, he chooses a statement rather than a request like *Can you charge it for me?* As before, he can't locate the words he needs to express his message, but he does a remarkably good job of finding a way to get the idea across. Val no doubt at first wonders what he means. Does he want the radio on while he shaves? But her knowledge of the context includes an awareness that the razor battery does go flat, and also that the razor makes a noise, which points her towards the correct interpretation.

What dementia does to communication

The description above reveals how much is going on in even a short conversation. But what you may have noticed is how very little of it is actually disorderly. In fact, the only real problem Val and Dad have

---

4   This process of reading between the lines is one aspect of *pragmatics*. An interesting discussion of the role of pragmatics in dementia communication is given by Guendouzi (2013).

is that Dad can't find the words for *razor* and *battery*. Everything else is a version of normal interaction.

But consider this. Suppose Val had been less patient with Dad when he mentioned sausages, throwing up her hands and saying *I don't know what you're talking about!* Suppose she'd assumed he was just being incoherent, rather than that he had a real goal of wanting to make a change in his world. She might never have found out what he needed, and he would have felt frustrated, defeated and, probably, hurt by her aggression or lack of interest in his needs.

Or suppose it hadn't been Val who was with him, but a professional carer who hardly knew him. The carer wouldn't have known that 'sausages' was his favourite substitute word and might have assumed he really did want sausages, or that he was hallucinating. She wouldn't necessarily have known that his razor ran on a rechargeable battery. She wouldn't have known where to go and find it. These are all elements of the context that Dad was relying on his listener knowing. If he'd been with someone without that information, the outcome would probably have been much less satisfactory. He wouldn't have got his message across and the carer wouldn't have met her goal of helping him.

We can now put those observations into the terms introduced in Chapter 2. Val's dad has, in Val, a high level of *social reserve*. As he falters on his route to shaving, she's there to hold him steady, like a parent holds the back of a child's bicycle saddle in those first stages of learning to ride. By supporting him with social reserve, she also protects his *emotional reserve*. People living with a dementia are very vulnerable to feeling frustrated, defeated and disappointed. But she signals to him that she cares about him, and that she wants him to achieve the changes in his world that he desires. This affirmation will set him up much better for the day ahead than negative emotions would.

Having explored Val and Dad's conversation in detail, we'll take a step back now, to look at the broader picture of how dementia creates challenges for communication. We already saw in Chapter 1 that dementia can upset the processes of producing and understanding sounds, words and grammar, and that topic will come up again in

Chapter 6. But next, we'll focus on the impact of not being able to track the context adequately, because this, in my view, lies at the heart of the daily challenges faced by people living with a dementia and those they interact with.

How problems with context-tracking undermine communication
Why context is so important

As we saw in Chapter 4, it's important to track the context during communication. That's because both the speaker and the listener need an accurate awareness of what the other does and doesn't know, believe and assume. When we communicate, we're usually trying to shift information into the zone of shared knowledge, as in Figure 5.1 – which is the same as Figure 4.3, except that there are now arrows, showing how information moves from the individual's knowledge into the zone of shared knowledge. To decide what we need to tell the other person, we must have an accurate awareness of what we both already know – what's in the shared zone already. And to judge what we can reasonably ask them to tell *us*, we need a good sense of what they know that isn't in the shared knowledge zone – after all, they can't be expected to tell us something they don't know.

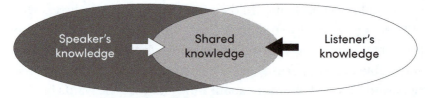

Figure 5.1: Shifting information into the zone of shared knowledge

For example, if I'm at the station and I want to know why the train's late, I'm likely to ask the platform guard. I'm judging that he knows and that he would be willing to move the information into the shared zone, so I know it too. Before he can reply, though, he may need some information from me that I falsely assumed was shared but actually wasn't – which train I'm referring to. Sometimes, we ask for or give information for other reasons as well. If I tell my colleague *It's my birthday today*, I probably didn't do it just so she knows when my birthday is. I might hope to change my world into one in which she gives me good wishes. If she then says *What are you doing for lunch?* then, again, she's not simply asking for information. She intends me to understand it as an invitation, given the contextual knowledge that is in the shared zone. And if I reply, *The Rose and Crown does very good steaks*, that wasn't a simple statement of fact either!

Taking all of this into account, we can see why problems arise if one of the participants in the conversation isn't able to process words quickly, pull together all the context or accurately calculate who knows what. In the first place, as a listener, they may not keep up with all the information that the speaker needs them to use. As a result, the assumptions a speaker makes about what a listener living with a dementia can work out from context may be unsafe. And then, when a person living with a dementia is the speaker, the judgements they make about the context information may not be complete or accurate. As a result, they could be assuming that the listener has more, less or different knowledge, than they actually do.

When speaker and listener can't make accurate guesses about what each other knows, it'll be difficult to communicate effectively. The less their beliefs about the context match up, the more risk there is that the listener won't interpret the message in the way the speaker intended. As a result, the speaker won't manage to get the changes they wanted to their world.

When people's contextual knowledge doesn't match up

A work colleague of mine recently described some contextual beliefs that her mother, living with a dementia, had:

> There were times when she thought the hospital ward was a brothel and the nurses were prostitutes. Another time, she was certain she was brought home from hospital in an open-backed lorry. During one stay in hospital she thought she had been left outside overnight.

What explains beliefs like this? Sometimes, dementia causes hallu-cinations. Sometimes, people living with a dementia interpret the sights and sounds around them as indicating a different situation from the one they're actually in. (Chapter 8 will consider what the options are for responding when this happens.) For instance, it's not uncommon for people living with a dementia who reside in a care home to believe they're in a hotel. We shouldn't be surprised about this particular misconception, because care homes and hotels have a lot in common. You have your own bedroom, while the other spaces, including a restaurant, are communal. There are other residents, whom you don't necessarily know. And there are staff whose job it is to clean your room, bring you food and drink, and generally ensure you are content.

If care homes were *exactly* like hotels, perhaps it wouldn't really matter if some residents didn't know which they were in. The prob-lems arise when a person's contextual assumptions are set up for one situation, and something happens that doesn't fit. The result can be confusion or indignation – for example, *Why are you telling me what time to go to bed, when I'm a guest here?* Overall, it would be surprising to find a care home resident whose belief that they were in a hotel didn't create some unease and disorientation at times.

Some dementia care environments go one step further, and actually encourage the residents to believe they're in a different context than the one they're really in. A notable example is the Hogeweyk dementia village in the Netherlands, designed to seem like an ordinary village with a shop, café, hairdressers and theatre, and with all the care staff appearing to just be village residents.[5] This deceptive environment is said to be highly beneficial to its residents, and Hogeweyk has been much praised for the quality of life it offers. But one can't help wondering whether residents sometimes sense that there's something not quite right about the place, and how that makes them feel. Chapter 8 will have more to say about Hogeweyk and other types of well-intentioned deceit of people living with a dementia.

---

5   https://hogeweyk.dementiavillage.com; see also Gallagher (2018)

It's likely, overall, that people living with a dementia become accustomed to coping with a rather hazy perception of where they are and what's going on and get used to not everything making total sense. But if they're to use communication to make changes to their world, then they do need to pin down enough contextual information to target their messages effectively. Dementia can interfere with the ability to recall information that was known earlier. It can also interfere with the processing necessary for taking in the information in the first place. When that happens, people living with a dementia may end up with less, or the wrong set of, contextual knowledge, compared with the person they're communicating with. Here are some of the things that they might, from time to time, not know or not be completely sure about:

- who they're talking with

- why they're having the conversation

- where they are

- what's going on around them

- what's already happened

- what's just been said

- what changes to their world are possible.

With such gaps in their knowledge of the context, people living with a dementia are at huge risk of making an error. They might address someone inappropriately because they thought they were someone else or had a different role. They might say something that's inappropriate for the situation, something that doesn't make sense or something that contradicts or repeats what's been said already. They might try to get others to make changes to their world that just aren't possible in that place or at that time.

Perhaps this wouldn't matter if those they were communicating with didn't have their own agendas and needs, but they do – we all do. If someone says something unexpected to us, we're likely to react quite strongly because it clashes with our own understanding of the context. It's disconcerting to come up against even small misalignments of contextual assumption. We might think, *But how CAN we do that?* and *Hang on, why is that relevant to EMILY?* and *I already TOLD you!* When a person living with a dementia doesn't have grasp of all the context we expect them to have, it's not only *their* communicative goals that are the likely casualties – it's ours as well.

Sometimes, context problems cause deep distress on both sides. Consider a person living with a dementia who one day doesn't recognize her son. She may well be embarrassed and upset when she's told who he is. Meanwhile, the son's entire world is anchored in his lifelong experience of the son–mother relationship. How can his mother *not* know who he is? And if she doesn't, what other beliefs that he's had up to now might also be wrong? Has she lost her grasp of the relationship because it was never important to her? If so, did his mother perhaps never really love him? In all events, does she love him now? How long has she not known who he was? Is this the end of the relationship they previously had? No wonder he's distressed.

Onward effects of context problems

All of this points to a major risk that there will be long-term effects for the person living with the dementia and/or those they communicate with – changes in basic behaviours. First, people living with a dementia may begin to realize that communicating is a hazardous business. Their attempts to change their world just don't tend to work. Repeated failure is no doubt frustrating and disappointing. The long-term risk is that they avoid going through all this unpleasantness by giving up trying to make changes to their world. Instead, they just put up with whatever situation they're in. They tolerate not knowing something, not enjoying something as much as they might, and so on. That's not a recipe for comfort or happiness, unfortunately.

Second, people living with a dementia can learn that the things they say seem to cause negative emotional reactions in other people, even though they didn't mean that to happen. For example, they discover that if they admit not recalling something, the other person becomes annoyed, frustrated or upset. Repeatedly getting such reactions from others will be uncomfortable and could cause guilt, confusion and anxiety. As a result, they may start modifying their behaviour to avoid the situation arising. They'll try to fit in with what others suggest, agree with what others say and not speak up when they aren't sure what's happening or have a different preference. In due course, they'll find their world is far from the way they'd really like it to be, and others may even stop asking them what they want.

Third, they may feel increasingly sad and frustrated that they're not able to play a role in others' lives. When someone tries to get them to help make a change in their own world, they're unable to respond, so they feel disappointed and useless. Fulfilling others' wishes is a way to keep our own world pleasant, because we like to feel useful and valued. The long-term risk for people living with a dementia is that they stop trying to respond to others' needs. It feels safer not to engage. And so we can find that people living with a dementia go quiet as a way of building a shield around their fragile emotions. To others, it will look as if they don't care, or aren't interested, when in fact they may have deep emotional needs that are not being met.

These different reactions are totally understandable in the circumstances, but they are clearly not good for the person's wellbeing. It'll be up to others around them to find ways to change the situation, so that these responses aren't necessary.

Ways to avoid the downward spiral

If we're to avoid creating the situations that could lead people living with a dementia to withdraw from communication, we need to notice what we might be doing that makes it likely to happen. We can't always stop our reactions, because we have our own important agendas and it's not surprising that we get frustrated if we can't achieve them. But our immediate emotional reactions are just that – they come out before we can take stock of how useful they are. If we start to notice what we're thinking and how we're feeling, we can gradually put just enough space between the event and how we react to it to make choices. Once we have choices, we can select responses that avoid making the situation worse.

For instance, if we say something and the person living with the dementia hasn't understood it, instead of getting frustrated, we can laugh and say, *Well, I didn't put that very clearly did I?* It doesn't matter whether it actually *was* clearly put or not – it obviously wasn't clear to them. By making a comment like that, we aren't blaming the person living with the dementia for not understanding. And that's good for their wellbeing. At the same time, although we're laying the fault at our own feet in a way, we're doing it with humour, so we aren't getting into self-blame (which it's important to avoid). And a good approach, to prevent us getting overwhelmed, is to see it all as an interesting project: *Let's see, how could I say this differently?* and *Hmm, I wonder why that didn't work well.*[6]

When people living with a dementia say something and we aren't sure what they meant, it's important to keep in mind that they had a purpose in speaking. They wanted some sort of response from us, whether an action, some information, acknowledgement or whatever. When we can't respond as they hoped, their world isn't getting changed as they wanted, which will be frustrating and disappointing for them. They didn't intend us to feel confused or annoyed by what they said. Nor did they intend us to feel guilty or anxious about not being able to understand *them*. So, even if what they've said causes some negative feelings in us, it's better just to notice them and move on. If those feelings persist, then it'll be helpful to find someone to talk them through with later, if possible.

Finally, if we notice that a person living with a dementia is becoming less willing to speak up for themselves, we can encourage them to express their preferences. This will help them rebuild confidence that it's worthwhile trying to change their world for the better. For example, it might work to offer them choices by *showing* them what the options are, rather than just mentioning them. And by encouraging them to talk about a topic that's easily within their grasp (such as reminiscences), we can help make their world into one where they're taken seriously and treated as interesting.

---

6   For a short film with ideas on how to approach communication difficulties as an interesting project, see Wray (2018).

Having seen how things can go wrong, in Chapter 6 we'll look at how, sometimes, solutions intended to compensate for a problem can make things worse.

ACTION POINTS FOR PEOPLE LIVING WITH A DEMENTIA

1. Think of a conversation where you didn't have enough information from the context to make sense of what was said. Did you or the other person manage to work out the problem? What could have been done better?

2. If there's a misunderstanding between you and someone else, what could the other person to do to help you? Could you suggest to them that seeing the funny side rather than getting frustrated is a good approach?

3. Have you noticed any particular places or situations that made you unsure what to do or say? Write them down or talk to someone about them. It might be possible to work out why it's particularly those places and situations that aren't giving you enough (or reliable) context information. For example, are they very busy, with lots of different things going on? Are they so plain that it's hard to get clues about where you are? Do they look like one thing, when in fact they're something else (for instance, a church turned into an art gallery)?

ACTION POINTS FOR FAMILIES, FRIENDS AND PROFESSIONALS

1. Reflect on conversations you've had with someone living with a dementia, where your beliefs about the context didn't match theirs and there was a misunderstanding. Looking back, what might you have done differently to get a more satisfactory outcome?

2. What places or situations seem to create most problems with context for the person living with a dementia that you know?

What is it about those situations? For example, is the person getting confused by a lot of coming and going? Are they looking for hints about the purpose of a place and not finding them? Are two different contexts interfering with each other (e.g. a concert given in a hospital, or a chance meeting with the dentist in the park)?

3. On a scale of 1–5, how easily do you get drawn into feeling frustrated, annoyed or upset when communication doesn't work well? Do you think the person living with the dementia realizes how you feel? What impact might it be having on them? (How would you feel in their shoes?) Is there anything simple you could do to change how you respond to these inevitable negative emotions?

ACTION POINTS FOR BYSTANDERS

1. When you interact with others in your daily work or life, do you tend to use jargon and specialist terms? Do you assume people know the terms and procedures in your domain? Have you ever had to explain things you thought were clear? This can be an issue even when the other person isn't living with a dementia. What might you do from now on so that people living with a dementia have the information they need when they deal with you?

2. Think of a time when there was a misunderstanding while communicating with a person living with a dementia. What happened and what did you do? Write a list of the different options someone in your position has in a situation like that (from walking away to painstakingly explaining everything). Judge which options on that list are practical and possible for you and start experimenting with them.

CHAPTER SIX

Those Awkward Moments

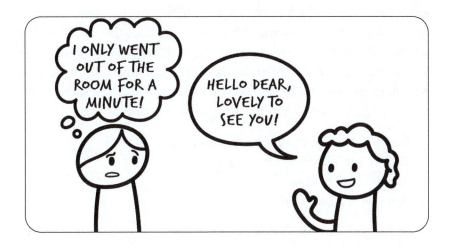

Bob's joke

In a TV documentary, *The Truth About Dementia*,[1] former newsreader Angela Rippon visited a married couple, Ida and Bob, who were long-standing friends of hers. Bob was living with Alzheimer's and Ida was his main carer. One particular scene stands out in my memory. It's Ida's birthday, and they're all sitting down for tea. The cake is cut, and then the following conversation takes place:

> *Angela: Happy birthday then, Ida, and many, many more, darling.*
> *Ida: Thank you. It's a lovely cake.*
> *Bob: Right, Merry Christmas.*

---

1   First broadcast on BBC Two on 19 May 2016.

Angela gives a quiet laugh. Bob laughs more loudly and lifts his slice of cake.
Angela: You've still got that to come.

What I find interesting about this conversation isn't so much what Bob says, but what Angela says in reply. It seems to me to be different from what she might have said to someone who wasn't living with a dementia. There's every indication that Bob's joking, and indeed Angela comments in the film immediately afterwards that 'the basic Bob', including his sense of humour, is still there. Nevertheless, Angela's comment looks like an attempt to 'tidy up' the context, so to speak. She's gently signalling to Bob that it's *not* Christmas. And this, we assume, is because she has some niggling doubt about whether he knows that fact or not. To understand why she might be unsure, we only have to look at what's previously happened. When Angela first arrives and greets Bob, the following conversation occurs:

Angela: Do you know it's her birthday today?
Bob: Whose birthday? Oh, Ida's?
Angela: Ida's birthday.
Bob: Oh yes, Ida's birthday, yeah.

Later, Ida goes out for a birthday treat on her own, while Angela stays with Bob. On her leaving, this exchange happens:

Ida: Come here.
Ida kisses Bob on the lips.
Angela: Is that her birthday kiss?
Ida: Is that my birthday kiss?
Bob: Is it your birthday today?
Ida pauses and says nothing.
Bob: Did I give you a present?
Ida: No.
Bob: Didn't I?

After Ida's return, they have lunch, starting with a toast to Ida:

Angela is pouring out sparkling wine.
Angela: There we go, Bob. Happy birthday to the birthday girl.

Ida: Thank you, Angela.
Ida, Bob and Angela clink glasses.
Bob: When's your birthday?
Ida: Today.

In short, Angela has had several indications that Bob isn't reliably retaining the information that it's Ida's birthday. Angela is protective towards Ida as well as Bob and has noticed that Ida seems upset when Bob doesn't recall her birthday. So, Angela is keeping a careful eye on what Bob's saying and why. It's not surprising she's uncertain whether his comment is a joke or a mistake.

Of course, *anyone* can say something we weren't expecting. How we resolve the clash depends on what we think caused it. When a professional comedian says something unexpected in a polished performance, we're very comfortable assuming it's a joke. If a child says, *There's a cow in the garden* and we know it's April Fool's Day, we'll guess it's a trick. But because Bob's living with Alzheimer's and has already indicated not recalling it's Ida's birthday, Angela can't be certain he's telling a joke, even though she knows he has a sense of humour. This leads her to say something she wouldn't need to say if she were certain Bob knew it wasn't Christmas.

In this chapter, I want to explore the nature and implications of this sort of uncertainty, because it has important effects on how we interact with people living with a dementia. How does it feel for a family member or professional carer who's constantly trying to juggle more than one possible interpretation of what might have been meant? And what's it like for a person living with a dementia when everything they say is being scrutinized for whether it's accurate and true?

To unwrap these issues, we'll look at some of the ways in which these awkward situations come about. One of them, ironically, is when someone tries to fix or anticipate communication problems. We'll then consider how such situations might be rescued, to save potential awkwardness and embarrassment.

Patching up problems

There are plenty of ways for communication to go awry when a person is living with a dementia. But there are also lots of ways for errors to get patched up. Sometimes, it's the person who doesn't have a dementia who tries to fix things – as we saw with Angela. But since many solutions are natural and automatic, it's often the person living with the dementia who fixes their own problem. We'll look at both sorts of fix here.

The kind of fix that's used depends, of course, on the problem. Chapter 5 showed how dementia can create difficulties in keeping up with the context (information about the world, including who's in the conversation and what's already been said and done). But, as we saw in Chapter 1, there are also some more basic challenges that dementia brings – in finding words and remaining fluent. So, we'll begin there.

When we're speaking, it's important to be reasonably fluent, otherwise people tend to interrupt us or lose interest. Unless we've got people's attention, it'll be impossible to get them to help us make changes to our world. To keep people's attention, we need to 'hold the floor'; that is, be the one speaking. As a result, we all have a range of tools we can use if we have a problem with fluency in our communication. These tools help us fix little blips and carry on talking. Even when we're not sure what we're trying to say, we have techniques to stop anyone else jumping in while we order our thoughts.

The most obvious and common tools are filler words and phrases like *um, er, you know, I mean*. But we see more extreme examples in, for instance, politicians' radio interviews, where they're keen not to let the interviewer cut in or pose a difficult question. Their tools include repeating themselves, repeating parts of what the other person said, and inserting stalling phrases like *I'm very glad you asked me that* and *Well of course that's a very interesting point you make there*, and so on, all of which can be produced more or less automatically, so the speaker can focus on working out what to say next.

People living with a dementia will naturally use the tools they've used throughout their lives, so we shouldn't be surprised to encounter expressions like *you know* and *I mean*, along with other phrases they've always had in their personal repertoire, such as *actually*, *in a manner of speaking*, *one way or another*, and so on. If they were previously good at filling in gaps by repeating themselves or stringing the sounds out to signal that they're in mid-thought, they may still do so. They may also develop new tools. One is *Pardon?*, which invites a repetition from the other person. This cleverly serves the dual purposes of buying time and giving them another go at understanding what was said to them, without fully handing over to the other person. Stock, or formulaic, phrases are often used to close off a bit of conversation when people aren't sure how to continue it. They might say, *Ah well, that's life* or *We shall see*.

Returning to the problem of not finding a word they need, people living with a dementia will sometimes replace the intended word with something else. It's not that this never happens to people without dementia, for we all occasionally say *Tuesday* when we meant *Wednesday* or *fridge* when we meant *washing machine*. But it's more common in dementia, and, as we saw with *sausages* for *razor* in Chapter 5, the replacements can be rather idiosyncratic. Many, if not most, replacements are completely automatic, rather than the speaker's choice, though words like *whatchamacallit* and *thingamajig* are more under our control.

Another solution when it's not possible to come up with a word is to judge how important the word actually is. It might be possible to move on without it. For example, one woman living with a dementia was telling a story and said, 'Let me try and see what was her name? I can't remember her name right now, uh gosh, well it doesn't matter about her name.'[2] Rather than holding up her story, she just ducked out of naming the person, so she could carry on.

Of course, it's particularly tricky if you can't recall the name of the person you're talking to. A colleague of mine told me how his uncle solved this problem. When anyone came into the room, he'd say, 'Hello, mate.' This meant he didn't need to come up with the name. When listeners notice that a person living with a dementia is struggling to recall names for things or people, they can often help

---

2 Ramanathan (1997, p. 46)

by inserting the information into their own message. For instance, if Jenny is telling a story, she might say, *And he said to me, 'Jenny, your cake is delicious.'*

In my study of Joan, the singing teacher introduced in Chapter 2,[3] I observed how good others were at filling in words that Joan wasn't able to come up with. Many times, it was David, the piano accompanist, who helped out. In the example below, Joan wanted to know whether the singer had sung the correct note, a B:

> **Joan:** *(She plays B several times on the piano) Are you, you know?*
> **David:** *Yes, she went right up to the B.*
> **Joan:** *Yes, that's right.*

On another occasion, one of the students provided a word:

> **Joan:** *She plays the trumpet in the what is it?*
> **Bella:** *The Guildhall.*
> **Joan:** *The Guildhall. She plays the trumpet at the Guildhall.*

The same occurs here, where we can also note one of Joan's empty filler phrases (she had several), *all the time*:

> **Joan:** *A little more of the... (she points to her own teeth)*
> **Kath:** *Teeth.*
> **Joan:** *Teeth, a little more of the teeth if you can do that all the time.*

The examples so far have illustrated how a fix is used after a problem arises. But both people living with a dementia and the people they communicate with sometimes anticipate problems that could arise in the future and take action in advance to avoid them. One of my neighbours, living with Alzheimer's, saw me in the street one day and I stopped for a chat with him. The first thing he said to me was, 'Now, I don't know if you know, but I've got Alzheimer's, and it means I can't remember people's names. I know who you are, but I don't know what you're called. I decided that I should tell people about my Alzheimer's so they would understand, and not be offended if I didn't know their name.'

---

3   Wray (2010)

This was a brilliant decision on his part. It meant it was impossible for me to be upset that he didn't recall my name. It also meant he didn't have to worry about hiding his difficulties. As a result, we were both much more relaxed as we chatted. I was even able to ask him how he was managing with his Alzheimer's, since he'd signalled awareness of his condition and willingness to talk about it.

Another example of pre-empting is saying something like *Sorry if I've said this before* or *I tend to repeat myself*. One counselling client of Danuta Lipinska's prepared a speech to deal with his tendency to say inappropriate things: 'I'm sorry if I say things that might be upsetting. I really don't know that I'm doing it and don't seem to be able to control it.'[4]

Other pre-emptive strategies include avoiding certain topics that might be difficult to discuss. For instance, it'll usually be harder to talk about objects and people that aren't present, because there's no opportunity to use gesture and touch as a substitute for the word. So, such topics might be set aside as too difficult.

Over time, there may be a temptation to pre-empt possible problems by letting someone who isn't living with a dementia speak on behalf of the person who is. It's common to find that a family member takes over in conversations with doctors or other professionals. We can see why. When time's short and it's vital to share important information, it may be the most effective approach. However, it's still important to ask the person's permission. It can be disempowering for the person living with the dementia to be represented rather than speaking for themselves. However, it could be a relief for them. In the following example, MB, living with a dementia, is keen to hand over responsibility to her daughter, when asked for information by the interviewer, MM:[5]

> *MM: How long were you in hospital? Were you there a lot?*
> *MB: Several times and – um you tell her. (addressed to her daughter)*

Finally, consider what Richard Taylor reports about dealing with the communication challenges associated with his Alzheimer's:

4   Lipinska (2009, p. 97)
5   Davis and Maclagan (2010, p. 206)

'I developed some pretty slick strategies to hide my scrambled and fading cognitive functions. I would control conversations, change subjects, use words few understand (and thus were hesitant to question) and on and on.'[6]

Unintended consequences

Because actual or potential communication glitches can be patched up, you can't always be sure if you're dealing with the problem itself or an attempt at a solution. Suppose a person living with a dementia greets his daughter with *Hello, mate* when she walks back into the room after a five-minute absence. How can the daughter tell if he doesn't recognize her, or if he's just using a catch-all greeting on her, even though he doesn't need to? The ambiguity can create the same kinds of awkward situation that we saw when Angela was responding to Bob's joke.

Consider the case of Bert and his late wife Nora, recounted to me by their granddaughter. Bert, living with a dementia, kept asking where Nora was. His family members gently explained that she was no longer alive, concerned that he'd be upset by this unexpected 'news'. But he became frustrated and agitated, telling them they were wrong. They tried to reason with him, but still he disagreed. In the end, he said, 'You know who I mean. She lives next door...with you!' He was referring to his daughter-in-law and had simply used the wrong name. He knew who he meant and he knew where she lived and with whom. This simple name substitution (a kind of automatic fix when the correct name didn't come to mind) made the entire situation seem quite different from what it was. Bert's family quickly jumped to the conclusion that the reason he'd mentioned Nora was because he'd forgotten she was dead. If Bert hadn't been living with Alzheimer's, they wouldn't have even contemplated that explanation This bias meant that they didn't really consider the possibility that he'd just produced the wrong name.

But that's not the end of the matter, because we have to consider

6   Taylor (2007, p. 138)

what might happen next time. Suppose on a later occasion Bert starts talking about 'Nora' again. The family has extra contextual information now. Whereas before they assumed he was referring to his wife, this time they have to consider the possibility that he's referring to his daughter-in-law, and his brain has solved the problem of not coming up with the correct name by using Nora's name instead. The problems is, they can't *know* that he is. He might, this time, actually mean his wife.

Situations like this mean the listener has to maintain two different possible interpretations in parallel. Until there's some clue that resolves the ambiguity, the entire rigmarole of tracking the context has to be doubled up. For example, if Bert mentions a holiday in Scotland with Nora, the listener needs to think about the holiday he took with his late wife *and* the one he took with his son and daughter-in-law. If he talks about how much he has always liked Nora's cooking, the listener must think about the dishes made by two women, instead of one. To manage this sort of ambiguity, they're likely to try to hedge their bets, keeping the whole range of interpretations alive. That means they must be vague in what they say in response, until they can get enough information to clarify what's meant. It's hard work, both because of the information that has to be managed, and because they're trying to deal with worries about making a false move and embarrassing themselves or the other person.

Let's extend the scenario another step. Suppose Bert pauses just at the point where he would have put in a name. Does that mean he's looking for the right name? Looking for the wrong name? Stopping because he realized he was about to come out with the wrong name and doesn't want to? And if so, does that indicate that he recalls having a problem in the past? Or has he paused for a quite different reason, such as changing his mind about what to ask? The irony is that the more Bert's family become aware that he might be using the wrong name or might not, the more possibilities they have to manage when trying to figure out how to proceed.

I imagine that most people who engage regularly with someone living with a dementia will be familiar with the experience of not knowing what to say next, because they're not quite sure whether the person meant to say what they just said. The same awkwardness must surely apply at times for people living with a dementia themselves. After all, some rather weird things must get said to them, and they have to figure out why. Let's consider an example of that.

Tina, living with Alzheimer's, and her husband Nick, were observed by Vai Ramanathan as part of her research into dementia communication.[7] Nick's approach when getting Tina to talk about her life was to ask her questions. However, they were questions to which he already knew the answer. For example, prompting Tina to talk about her father, he asked, 'When did he die, Tina?' and 'How did he die?' We don't usually ask questions that provide us with no additional information, and if we want to hear something we already know, we'd say something like *Tell me again how he died*, with the implication that hearing the story again might give us some new information.

Using the model of communication presented in Chapter 3, we have to ask ourselves what Nick was trying to achieve. What did he want Tina to do on his behalf, that would improve his world? Clearly, it wasn't shifting information that only she had into the shared zone of knowledge (Chapter 5, Figure 5.1). His purpose must have been simply to get her to talk. This is entirely reasonable, particularly since there was a researcher present. And in fact his approach for achieving his goal worked quite well, for she did indeed recount stories from her childhood in response to these prompts. That's not the issue. The issue is that unless she was able to appreciate his purpose, it must have seemed quite odd to her to be asked these apparently information-seeking questions by someone she knew had that information already. In a nutshell, Nick's attempts to help her solve her communication problems created a rather strange situation that could have increased her cognitive load and/or anxiety.

Strange situations can also occur when the communication is simplified in order to help people living with a dementia. For example, suppose that in a care facility there are two main options at dinner time (say, roast chicken and fish pie today), plus a range of alternatives that are always available (such as omelette, jacket potato

---

7   Ramanathan (1997, pp. 82–87)

and pasta with cheese). The staff are aware that listing the full range of choices is overwhelming for some residents, and so, for those individuals, the staff bring out two plates, one with each main option on, and invite the person to point to the one they would prefer. This is a sensible and effective solution to the difficult challenge of finding out what the person would like to eat.

However, it might also be rather confusing for the resident to only be offered a choice between fish pie and chicken, when it's clear that some people are eating jacket potatoes, omelettes and pasta. Not only might they have preferred one of those options, they may not be able to fathom how you get them. This is because they have been put, albeit for understandable reasons, into a situation where those other options aren't on offer. They might fret about why they're not allowed those other things. Is it a punishment? Did they say or do something that took those choices away?

In summary, there's a risk that the attempt to patch up communication problems introduces problems of its own, for the person living with the dementia, the person they are communicating with, or both. Any underlying problem can potentially be tackled in many different ways and, conversely, what a person says on a given occasion could potentially be the result of trying to deal with several different problems. Not surprisingly, anyone in the conversation could become anxious: *Will I be able to follow what's said? Will it be clear what is meant? Will I know how to respond without embarrassing myself or the other person?*

Importantly, these awkward situations come about as a result of people's ability to hold different understandings of the situation in balance. In other words, the more insight someone has, the more challenges they'll be dealing with.

There's yet one more unintended consequence to be mentioned, and this, too, arises from being good at appreciating the complexity of the situation. We saw in Chapter 5 how important it is to keep track of the context if communication is to be effective. We also saw how context tracking can go wrong when people living with a dementia don't have the level of contextual knowledge that the other person in the conversation assumes they do.

If neither party has much capacity to see things from the other person's perspective, there's likely to be a clash – confusion and frustration are the most common outcomes. But if we become aware that people living with a dementia have too little contextual information or have a different belief about what contextual information is relevant, then our own job becomes more complicated. In addition to following our *own* contextual information, we need to try keeping track of what the other person's is like and decide how to take it into account. Here's an example.

In an interview on the BBC radio programme *Broadcasting House*,[8] Sue talked about her husband Trevor, who was living with a dementia. He was a former policeman and sometimes now believed he was back at work, rather than in a residential home. Sue described how she had to go along with him, if he thought he was at work:

> Very often, we're in the police station and we're charging goodness knows how many criminals and we're weighed down with stuff and we have to get on with it, so this is how the conversation goes, and I just carry on with it. 'Yes, okay, Trev, I'll be along later, and just send the stuff to me and I'll get it back to you.' And then he's happy and that's the way it goes. And I have to laugh because I know he's in his own little world, and he's not fretting for me.

Sue's juggling several things at once here. First, she has to keep a grip on the context as *she* sees it: where she is, what's happening, and why. She'll be constantly aware that Trevor is living with a dementia, and that, as a result, he sometimes doesn't share as much of her knowledge of the situation as she might expect. This is part of the context within which she makes decisions about her own communication. For instance, on account of his current beliefs, she might decide *not* to try to get Trevor's help in changing some aspect of her own world (such as getting comfort from him if she's distressed). Instead she might approach a staff member in his care home, or just suppress the desire for that change entirely.

Second, part of her contextual knowledge is the experience she's

---

8   Broadcast on BBC Radio 4 on 26 July 2020.

built up over time. That experience might tell her that Trevor will be most content if she buys into his beliefs rather than challenging them.[9] To do that, she has to work out what he believes and operate within that world. For instance, he has assigned particular roles to different people around him: some are fellow police officers, some are administrative staff, some are criminals. Only by seeing his world as he sees it can she avoid saying or doing something that doesn't match his expectations – leading to anxiety or frustration. So, she needs to be attentive to what he says and does and use those observations to enrich an add-on context that's temporarily part of *her* world.

Anything she says to him will need to be driven by that add-on context, because that's the one he shares with her. So, if she wants to change her world into one where he's sitting quietly with a cup of tea, for instance, she'll need to step inside his world to do so. She might tell him that the sergeant says it's time for his tea break. Meanwhile, if Trevor's world leads him to do something that isn't acceptable in Sue's and the staff's context, they'll need to use *his* world to sort it out. For example, if he tries to use force to 'arrest' someone or tries to leave the building to attend a crime scene, those around him will need to guide him, within his context, away from these actions into other actions that are more acceptable to them but still make sense to him. If that sounds complicated, it's because it is. It's cognitively tiring, and some people also find it emotionally and ethically challenging. For, as we'll see in Chapter 8, there's been considerable debate about whether it's a good or bad thing to buy into the false beliefs of people living with a dementia.

The most challenging type of clash between contextual worlds occurs when people living with a dementia want to go home to their (long-dead) mother and father, or are anxious about having abandoned their (actually grown-up) young children, due home from school. It'll be necessary to seek out and address the deeper needs that such longings arise from, such as a sense of abandonment, a need for comfort or a desire to be important to someone. Once again, a sort of mental gymnastics is required, to think behind what's said

---

9   For more on this topic, see Chapter 8.

and figure out what change to the person's world is really needed. In the next section, we'll look at how these situations are best approached, to maximize the wellbeing of all concerned.

Resolving awkward moments and their associated challenges

We've seen so far the complex paths that can lead to confusion, awkwardness and the need to balance contradictory information. We've also had a hint of the immediate solutions that can be tried. At a more general level, there are some principles that can assist us when dealing with these situations.

Principle 1: Learn to tolerate ambiguity and uncertainty

An important first step is recognizing that you often won't know enough to make the perfect judgement about how to respond. When two people share less contextual knowledge than they expected (irrespective of whether one of them is living with a dementia), there will be false assumptions and expectations and, inevitably, confusion. It's only a question of whether that develops into anxiety, annoyance, frustration, and so on. You can't control the uncertainty, but you do have a measure of control over how you react to it – with positive or negative effects on the feelings of the person living with the dementia.

Principle 2: Approach the situation with compassion and kindness

We can find it difficult to manage situations calmly and benevolently when our expectations and beliefs tell us that things ought to be different from how they are. On the other hand, when we don't have any particular expectations about a person or a situation, it's often much easier to be practical, creative and compassionate. That's why it can be less stressful to help a person living with a dementia if they're a stranger than if they're a family member. As a family member, we have a long history of expectations and assumptions and it's sometimes hard to let them go. Standing back from our immediate emotional involvement can help us keep perspective and retain choice about how we react. Then we can more easily access our capacity to act with understanding and kindness.

Principle 3: Be alert for clues and treat the mysteries with interest and fun

Dementia takes people – both those with the diagnosis and those around them – on a journey. We might as well look around us, notice the new landscapes and learn from what we experience. Treating the experience of engaging with a person living with a dementia as intriguing and interesting can help it seem less overwhelming. If something goes wrong, it's often more helpful to be curious about what happened and how things might be done differently next time, than to succumb to despondency, frustration or guilt.

Principle 4: Be adaptable and go with the flow

Tancredi, a character in Lampedusa's novel *The Leopard*, famously comments: 'If we want things to stay as they are, things will have to change.'[10] There's a risk that in trying not to lose the person beneath the dementia, we grab onto the wrong things. We'd like the person to continue doing and saying the things they used to. We'd also like them to be content in themselves. But if both are not possible, which is it better to prioritize? Forcing someone to continue behaving in ways that are no longer easy or natural for them means we're not accepting that they're changing. We may make them unhappy by not accepting these alterations.

Regularly taking stock of where things are, what's changed and what hasn't can help ensure that the person living with the dementia is accepted for who they now are and allowed to have the preferences

---

10 Lampedusa (1958/2007, p. 19)

and opinions they now have. At the same time, it will help us see more clearly what we most want to help the person hold on to, so it doesn't change sooner than it needs to.

Trevor's wife, Sue, quoted earlier, recounts what he said to her after the Covid-19 lockdown in spring 2020 had kept them apart for several weeks:

> He told me that he'd got married. He said, 'I can't go on like this.' He said, 'I got married yesterday.' And I said, 'Oh, did you?' 'Yes,' he said, 'she's a very nice lady, she lives in this place, and I thought I'd get married again.' So I said, 'Well, what about me?' So he said, 'Well, I think there's something like an annulment that you can get,' and I said, 'Well I don't want an annulment, Trevor, I love you, and you're my husband,' and he went, 'Oh, well, alright then, okay, I'll tell her, I'll tell her to go. But it was a nice service.' (She laughs). So that's when I knew there might be a chance he was forgetting me.

Sue shows us here that she's found a way to accept and work with what Trevor tells her, without getting it out of proportion. She uses her conversation with him to bring him into line with the most important part of her own reality – that they're still married. In terms of the communication model in Chapter 4, she knows what she wants to achieve: that he acknowledges being her husband. She uses as her starting point her own understanding of the situation, which includes the nature of his disease. Then, she takes note of the claims he's making. These claims signal to her how he sees things at the moment and form the basis of the knowledge she shares with him (even though she doesn't agree with it) – that he's married someone else. From there, by saying she doesn't want an annulment, that she loves him and that she wants to stay married to him, she introduces information into the shared zone that he doesn't (appear to) have. Her approach is successful in getting him to acknowledge this (new) information, which is what she was aiming for.

Principle 5: Identify battles that you're fighting unnecessarily

What Sue's approach shows us is that if we want to achieve changes to our world, and the person who'll help us make them is living with a dementia, we need to find a starting point that they can relate to. Importantly, we also need to take a long hard look at what changes we want them to help us make, and only try for ones that can succeed. Sue doesn't ask Trevor to apologize for claiming to have deserted her. She doesn't try to get answers from him about who this other woman is. She doesn't try to explain that the reason she seemed to desert him was the Covid-19 lockdown. She understands the bigger picture and takes control of her situation by making choices.

ACTION POINTS FOR PEOPLE LIVING WITH A DEMENTIA

1. You're probably aware that sometimes the effects of your dementia cause awkwardness for yourself or others. Have you considered getting in first, by explaining your condition to people?

2. Experiment with laughing and saying *Oops!* when something goes wrong in a conversation. It can be remarkably effective. It's hard for someone to be frustrated if the slip is acknowledged. Then you can jointly work out how to get the message across.

3. How do you feel about people speaking on your behalf in conversations with others? Perhaps you could discuss with people close to you whether you mind being sidelined and how you'd like them to involve you.

ACTION POINTS FOR FAMILIES, FRIENDS AND PROFESSIONALS

1. How quickly do you cut in and talk on someone's behalf? Have you checked (by asking them or observing them) whether they

mind? Given that you may have good reason to assist in some situations (e.g. with a doctor or other professional), how could you ensure that what you say will be representative of what the person living with the dementia would say for themselves?

2. Have you experienced situations when you didn't know what to say, because you weren't sure what the person living with the dementia meant? Next time it happens, try to notice how you feel. Can you judge how they feel? What could break the awkwardness? For instance, would it work if you (or the other person) laughed and said, *I've no idea what just happened!*

3. How adaptable do you think you are to the changing situation caused by the person's dementia? List the things you most want to hold on to and the things you don't mind losing. For instance, how much do you mind if they can't recall the name of the dog? How about if they can't recall your name? Although you can't control how things change, you can control what you care about, and that will give you more energy to assist the person in retaining the information and behaviours that matter to you most. Discussing these ideas with (other) family members could help them adapt too.

ACTION POINTS FOR BYSTANDERS

1. Have you observed a family member or carer speaking on behalf of the person living with a dementia? Even if it's more convenient for you, be sensitive to the potential effect. If it seems to be causing frustration or distress, try to involve the person living with the dementia more.

2. Family and professional carers who spend a lot of time with people living with a dementia can sometimes find it hard to see alternative ways of handling situations. As a bystander, you may be in a stronger position to notice opportunities for alternatives. Experiment with them, as this may raise others' awareness of these options.

CHAPTER SEVEN

Does Dementia Change Someone into a Different Person?

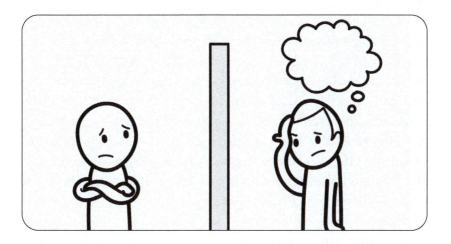

Iris and her carer

In an investigation of dementia carers' 'emotional labour' (the effort involved in managing our emotions), Simon Bailey and colleagues[1] showed how residential care staff try to keep a balance between two competing priorities – understanding the feelings and predicament of people living with a dementia on the one hand and, on the other, keeping enough emotional detachment to get the practical jobs done.

---

1 Bailey et al. (2015)

In that study, one carer reported a conversation he'd had with Iris, a resident living with a dementia. Iris had recently moved from a different ward, where she'd been considered difficult to manage. Iris explained that staff had made her angry by trying to force her to eat and take her medication. She felt their treatment had made her behave out of character and she was unhappy about getting this unjust reputation. This is what the carer said about that conversation:

> To me, the fact that she not only remembered events of a few weeks back but was also capable of thinking rationally about the nature of her behaviour and the reaction to it by the staff was oddly disconcerting. One of the ways that I feel able to keep a positive outlook towards many of the patients' emotional states is through the reassurance that they don't really seem to know what is going on.[2]

The carer's comment shines a light on an important aspect of how people living with a dementia are often viewed and treated. To do his job, the carer needed to protect himself emotionally (i.e. keep a reasonable level of emotional reserve for himself, see Chapter 2). To do that, he'd categorized Iris and his other clients as *different* from unimpaired people ('they don't really seem to know what is going on'). That allowed him to avoid getting too sad about their situation. Discovering that Iris actually wasn't different in that way concerned him, because it meant he'd misjudged her ability to understand the frustrations and indignities of her situation.

This chapter considers whether it's valid and useful to view people living with a dementia as different – different from those without dementia, and different from the person they used to be. If it is, where and when do they cross that line? What consequences are there of having such a divide and where it's placed? It turns out to be a complicated matter.

---

2   Bailey et al. (2015, p. 262)

What counts as 'different'?

In a moving unpublished account of his experience of caring for his wife who's living with a dementia, David Green writes:

> I've only ever had one marriage, but somehow I seem to have acquired a second wife... Although I still catch glimpses of my first wife, she doesn't linger. Gradually my new wife is taking over. Thankfully, thus far, she does seem to share some of the lovely nature that my first wife possessed.[3]

What he's describing is not a sudden change in his wife into someone different from before, but something much more gradual and subtle. For this reason, we need to abandon the stark contrast between *same* and *different*. Dementia is one of many life events that obviously do change people, including ageing, getting married, having a child, changing job, giving up smoking, and so on. So the real questions are: *How and to what extent is someone changed by dementia?* and *How do others look on those changes?*

In my previous work, I've proposed an alternative approach to understanding the changes caused by dementia. It involves recognizing that there are differences, but viewing them as differences of either *degree* or *kind*.[4]

People who are different in *degree* from how they were before, and from people who aren't living with a dementia, have changed, but only in the sense that some characteristics are a little more extreme. For example, they might be a bit more forgetful than other people, or a bit more anxious. The characteristics that have changed are on a continuum – behaviours and experiences that everyone has, albeit to a lesser extent. When viewed this way, the effects of dementia are no different from, say, becoming a little more unsteady on our feet as we get older, or having a smaller appetite than before.

Richard Taylor captures the situation in the following: 'Physicians, friends and family are forever asking me, *How is it going? Do you still feel okay? Having any problems?* The measures used to

---

3   David Green, Reflections of a dementia carer' (unpublished notes), personal communication
4   Wray (2020b, chapter 10)

evaluate my answers seem to grow from the unstated question, *Are you still like me?*[5]

In contrast, when someone's viewed as different in *kind*, there's a firm divide between how they are now and how they used to be, or how they are and how others are. For example, a person living with a dementia might swear when they never did before, or they might be violent when they used not to be. If they can't recognize their loved ones, this too may suggest that they've crossed a line and are no longer the same person they once were. The characteristics that suggest a person is different in kind are ones that strike others as unusual, abnormal and difficult to empathize with. We might find it impossible to imagine looking at our own child and thinking they were a stranger, or what it would be like to have completely changed our personality.

But our judgements about others may not always be reliable. At the start of this chapter, we saw how Iris was labelled by her carer as different in *kind* because he assumed she didn't really know what was happening to her. Her account of how she'd been treated in her last ward shocked the carer as he realized she was much more like him than he'd thought – different only in *degree* – for she was able to recall past events and reflect on them. We, reading the story, may also recognize how like us she is – wouldn't we also get angry if someone tried to make us eat and take medication when we didn't want to?

Two things probably seem obvious at this point. One is that it's more humane to view someone living with a dementia as being different in degree than different in kind. The other is that as a person's dementia develops over time, there'll be a shift in one direction only: from being perceived as different in degree towards being perceived as different in kind. Both these observations are true to an extent, but I'll show presently that it's not quite as simple as it looks.

---

5   Taylor (2007, p. 176)

The pros and cons of difference in degree and kind
Empathy

The major advantage of seeing someone as different from oneself only in *degree* is that it's easier to have empathy. We have empathy when we can understand how someone feels. We can only understand how they feel if we can identify how we're similar to them.

A few years ago, I was in a large supermarket with a café on the floor above. I decided to have a cup of tea and so went up the escalator. When I was ready to leave, I discovered that the down escalator was broken and a staff member was directing people to the lift. This wasn't a problem for me, but during the descent, I could see that one person was looking very uncomfortable. As soon as the doors opened, he rushed out ahead of everyone else. I went after him and asked if he was okay. He explained that he got panic attacks in lifts and had hated being forced to use one. I noticed two reactions in myself, when given this information. My first reaction was to think: *We were only in the lift a few seconds, so how could you get that panicky? After all, I wouldn't.* This is a sort of empathy in that I was thinking about what I'd feel like in his situation. However, it wasn't all that helpful, because I'd never had the experience of getting claustrophobic in a very short lift journey. Although I was 'putting myself in his shoes', it was still *myself* I was focusing on. We can call this approach *self-based empathy*.

But then a different perception came into my head. It was a reversal of how I'd seen things before. Instead of somehow doubting his experience because it didn't match mine, I thought: *What would it take for me to feel that panicky?* This put me in mind of experiences I'd had on parapets at the top of high buildings. By drawing on those experiences, I could fully understand how terrible he felt. Different things triggered the feelings in him compared with me, but that was irrelevant. What mattered was connecting the feelings. We can call this *response-based empathy*.

It's impossible for those of us not living with a dementia to understand what it feels like for people who are, so self-based empathy can't get us very far. But response-based empathy can. Let's explore this by thinking about a person living with a dementia who keeps asking the same question over and over again. With self-based empathy we might think, *If I were in your shoes, I'd concentrate a bit harder, or write the answer down if I thought I wasn't going to recall it.* But in response-based empathy we might think, *What would it take for me to be so anxious about something that I had to keep asking about it?* We might be able to recall some situation when the information we were given didn't put our mind at rest. For instance, at a railway station once, I became fairly sure that the platform I'd been directed to wasn't the right one. I kept checking the display boards and asking people. The platform was correct, I was told. However, I remained worried because I knew I'd struggle to get to another platform with my heavy luggage if there was a last-minute announcement to cross the footbridge (which, as it turned out, there was). Recalling that experience helps me understand what a person living with dementia might feel like if they weren't sure they had all the information they needed.

Response-based empathy makes us more likely to come up with appropriate actions to help the person. At the station, it wouldn't have been enough for someone to say, *Stop worrying, this is the right platform!* Whoever was right, I wasn't going to feel comfortable until I was on the train *and* I'd become calm again. In the same way, if a person living with a dementia is asking the same question repeatedly, we need to recognize that getting the answer might not be enough. There may be an underlying anxiety that needs to be resolved, and they may also need some kindness from us before they feel okay.

The response-based approach to empathy opens the way for people living with a dementia to be treated as humanely as possible, and that gives it a major advantage over viewing someone as different in degree. However, there are also some snags with *different in degree* that can be resolved by switching to the *different in kind* viewpoint.

Self-protection

When we see a person living with a dementia as different from us only in *degree*, we'll try to interpret everything they say and do as a version, albeit more extreme, of something we might do ourselves.

And that can create a problem for us. Dementia is a frightening prospect. Most people are nervous about developing anything that might be an early sign of dementia. As a result, we can find it very disturbing to see a person living with a dementia as someone who's just got a little bit further down the same path that we're on. It's a lot more comforting to draw a stark line between ourselves and those living with a dementia. We might think, *This person's very forgetful. Okay, I know I'm sometimes forgetful, but my forgetfulness is definitely not like theirs. So, mine doesn't indicate that I'm developing a dementia.* Or, *This person repeats anecdotes quite often. All right, I know I occasionally tell the same story more than once, but that's different!*

When we put up these barriers, we're moving away from the *different in degree* viewpoint towards *different in kind*. But it's very understandable. It's a way of coping with the uncertainties of life, and it's particularly attractive to people who live or regularly work with someone living with a dementia. They can protect their emotional reserve (to an extent) by not identifying too closely with them.

Drawing a line so the person living with the dementia is seen as different in kind can help in another way as well. Sometimes, a person's dementia can cause them to say things that are potentially hurtful or unappreciative. They might not show affection towards a close relative who desperately needs that reward and recognition. They might be aggressive, even violent. If the person is viewed as different only in degree, then their behaviours have to be interpreted in the same way as if they weren't living with a dementia. That means a hurtful comment was made on purpose. In contrast, if the person is viewed as different in kind, then all bets are off. They won't be expected to behave in the same way as others. The dementia can explain and excuse their behaviour. This is one of the potential advantages of adopting the *different in kind* position.

Inhumane treatment

So far, then, we've seen that viewing someone as different in degree enables us to have empathy, but also makes us more vulnerable to being hurt. Seeing someone as different in kind means we can keep some emotional distance. The risks, however, are significant. If someone is different in kind, then carers and others are less likely to base their treatment of the person on how they'd want to be treated themselves. Instead, they'll be looking at the person from the outside, with little attention to how it feels to be treated that way, and what the person wants and prefers.[6] That's how we get 'care' that's not really caring at all. David Clegg reports observing the following incident in a residential care home for people living with a dementia. Daisy, one of the residents, is singing loudly:

> A carer comes and puts on a CD and turns it up in order to drown out Daisy's singing. After a few seconds the CD sticks. The carer leaves the room with the CD repeating the same tiny fragment of music.[7]

The act of leaving the CD on repeat appears to be a 'punishment' for Daisy, without any consideration of the experience that she, or any of the other residents around her, would have as a result. Such behaviour is not humane.

The media often report even more inhumane treatment of people living with a dementia – hitting them, restraining them or leaving them alone, dirty and underfed. This, as Kitwood notes, 'turn[s] those who have dementia into a different species, not persons in the full sense'.[8] Athena McLean, who compared the approach to care in two wards in the same nursing home (one ward was much more humane than the other), describes how, in the less humane ward, care was 'something that was done *to* a person, like a procedure to an object'.[9]

It's easy, and appropriate, to call out such bad treatment, but Clegg points out that we need to have some empathy for the carers as well:

> Although the carers cannot be freed from their direct responsibility for the abuses...it is important to see that they too were trapped in a faulty system. Each person was being asked to cope with long

---

6   Wray (2020b, p. 212)
7   Clegg (2010, p. xxx)
8   Kitwood (1997, p. 14). In keeping with the suggestions in this chapter, he refers to it as 'a highly defensive tactic' – that is, not due to intentional unkindness but rather an attempt to cope.
9   McLean (2007, p. 198)

hours or unpleasant, hot, smelly, tiring work and occasional acts of physical violence with little reward. Most had started the job with good intentions and they as much as [the residents] had been failed by low staffing levels, paltry activities budgets, unimaginative training and little understanding of their own need for support or praise for their efforts.[10]

In short, if we're to promote approaches that support the wellbeing of people living with a dementia, it can't be done by simply criticizing those who treat them as different in *kind*. We need to recognize why they do so and explore how to help them find alternative ways of seeing things.

Anxiety

Finally, it's important, though emotionally challenging, to consider how people living with a dementia view each other. Imagine a person living with moderate dementia symptoms encountering someone whose dementia has progressed to the stage where they shout, are aggressive and don't understand where they are or what's happening. The person living with moderate dementia will be aware that dementia gets worse over time, and they might fear one day being similarly confused and distressed. Rather than seeing the person with advanced dementia as different in kind (which would be emotionally safer), they start to see them as different only in degree – like themselves, except a bit further down the track. This issue is rarely talked about but it's important because of the anxiety it's likely to cause. We can help by treating all people living with a dementia as being like us, and essentially the same as they ever were, whenever possible. This will help those with moderate dementia feel anchored into a normal life and also reassure them that even if their symptoms do get worse, they will be treated with care and empathy.

---

10   Clegg (2010, p. iii)

An alternative way of thinking about degree and kind

So far, I've talked about how people get viewed and treated as different in *degree* or in *kind*. However, that simple two-way perspective is far too limited. So I now want to suggest some modifications to that approach that can bring us closer to identifying ways of supporting people living with a dementia better.

The first modification is to acknowledge that people vary – from situation to situation and day to day – in how far they're a version of their old self and/or of the population generally, and how far they're different in kind from that. Allowing for variation reduces the risk that someone gets permanently viewed as different in kind because of one thing they did one day. After all, not bringing their grandchild's name to mind today doesn't mean they might not do so tomorrow.

The second modification is recognizing that people might be at different points along the continuum for different abilities. Figure 7.1 shows how that might look for a particular individual with mid- to late-stage dementia. Note that this is illustrative only. Each person will have their own version of these balances. So the description that follows isn't an attempt to characterize everyone's dementia at a given stage, just to illustrate one person's experience of living with their particular dementia.

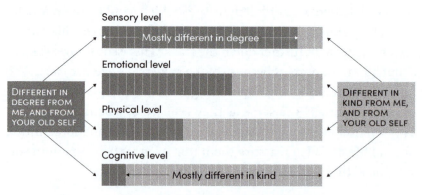

Figure 7.1: Degree–kind continuums for different functions

If we begin from the bottom of Figure 7.1, we see that the person's cognitive abilities (memory, concentration, ability to take in new information, work things out, produce and understand language, and so on) have deteriorated to a considerable extent. It's quite hard for family and professionals to directly relate to the person's experiences. As indicated in the diagram by the light-coloured gradations outnumbering the dark ones, for these abilities, the person is largely, though not entirely, viewed as being different in *kind*. This means they're not really expected to be able to perform at the same level as an unimpaired person. They won't be asked to do things that require them to remember lots of information, and they might not be left for long on their own.

At the next level up in the figure, we see that physically, the person is somewhat impaired, but not as badly as with cognition. Maybe they can walk around indoors, provided they use a walking aid, but need assistance to go to the toilet, and would be at risk outside, because of the hazards of uneven ground or busy traffic. Family and professionals can view the person as different in *degree* for some activities, such as helping fold the washing, preparing vegetables and changing the TV channel. This means the person is assumed able to do the task and is trusted to do it more or less as anyone else would, albeit a little more slowly or with a bit less finesse. Meanwhile, other physical activities need to be supervised, or aren't offered to the person at all, because for these, they're viewed as different in *kind*. They're considered 'not the sort' to be able to do them alone. For example, a family member might say, *Oh, I don't think you should mow the lawn any more,* or *I don't want you going in the shower without me around.*

Moving up another level in Figure 7.1, we see that emotionally speaking, the person has not moved as far along the continuum and is still primarily viewed as different in *degree*. This means they're generally expected to respond emotionally like anyone else. For instance, they're still funny, kind, grateful, interested, and so on – or perhaps still as annoying, cantankerous and mean as they used to be! Being at this place on the continuum means more's expected of them, though. They're assumed to be taking responsibility for how they behave towards others and they'd be expected to pick up on someone else's anxiety or sadness and respond appropriately, like anyone else would. If they don't, then the family member will be hurt by what will seem to be a deliberate lack of concern. Only at a later point, when the person's considered to have moved much further along the continuum, will such a failure to respond be forgiven as *only to be expected from someone who's not like me*, or *not like their old self*.

All the same, the emotion continuum in Figure 7.1 is also already part-way to *different in kind*. That might be because the person's emotional responses are less 'normal' at certain times of day, or when something unexpected happens. It's part of the job of family and professional carers to get to know which sorts of events might trigger the changes in a person's responses that potentially move them into the zone where they're different to others and to their pre-dementia self.

The top level in Figure 7.1 relates to the person's sensory abilities – their sight, hearing, touch, smell and taste. Here, the person is largely treated like anyone else – different only in *degree*. They're slightly less able to see clearly, and/or slightly hard of hearing, say, but nothing that's at odds with many other people. They still enjoy being hugged and still love the taste of fresh raspberries and cream. Importantly, this is a major means by which family and professionals can feel confident of reaching them. If all else fails (conversation's difficult, for example), they know the person will value having their hand held. For completeness, though, let's consider that small zone at the *different in kind* end on the sensory continuum. The person might report that a lot of foods taste 'greasy'. This would be hard for others to imagine or accommodate – so the person is, in that respect, viewed as rather 'odd' and 'abnormal'.

Deciding when to view a person as different in kind

It may have become clear to you while reading the previous section that even within one of those ability levels there are likely to be differences in where on the continuum someone is. As just noted for sensory abilities, someone could be seen as different in degree for sight and hearing, but different in kind for taste. Similarly, on the cognition continuum, someone could be different in degree when it comes to talking about knitting and sewing, but different in kind in conversations that call on recent memory. This makes it even more important to avoid assuming that someone is completely unable to experience life like other people can, and as they used to in the past.

With regard to cognitive abilities, one important focus of interest is the *capacity to make decisions*. Figure 7.1 helps us understand why it's rarely as simple as saying that a person *does* or *doesn't* have the capacity to contribute to decision-making about their own life. In each situation, an assessment should be made about whether the person understands the issue and can take into account sufficient relevant information. It's important to accommodate their best interests by being flexible.[11] One opportunity for flexibility is to take into account how high the stakes are on this particular occasion. It might be judged risky to let the person make a binding legal decision without support and guidance. But there's no reason not to let them choose which jigsaw puzzle they do next or which room they'd prefer if they move into residential care.

The more opportunities people living with a dementia have to exercise their capacity for decision-making, the more we'll see them as different only in *degree*, with onward benefits for appropriate and sensitive treatment. However, in the real world, there is a significant risk that this doesn't happen, and a person gets permanently viewed as different in *kind*. Although we've seen that a *different in kind* approach can be helpful and beneficial in some circumstances, overall it's not a good thing if that view becomes dominant.

Getting stuck in *different in kind* is what Tom Kitwood termed 'malignant social psychology',[12] which leads to hostile behaviour. Kitwood identifies 17 such behaviours, including being patronizing, not accepting the person's point of view, mocking them, treating them like an object rather than a human being and labelling them in ways that overlook important aspects of the whole person.

Poor communication is a major potential trigger for people living with a dementia getting stuck with the *different in kind* label. That's because, as we've seen in the previous chapters, we all respond very strongly to not achieving what we intended to through our

---

11   My thanks to Pauline Strong for this important observation.
12   Kitwood (1997, p. 14)

communication. We can only achieve our goals if the other person is able to pick up on our message and respond appropriately. People living with a dementia are less able to do that, with the result that they can get sidelined as incapable of participating in communication in a useful way.

Meanwhile, people living with a dementia also struggle to achieve their own goals, because they can't set up the messages in quite the way that the other person expects. As they increasingly fail to achieve effective communication, they may try less often, and it will be easy for others to write them off as not needing or wanting to make changes to their world. It's another way in which they can seem to be different in kind. That, however, is a very damaging assumption to make:

> Unless we believe that people living with a dementia are one hundred percent content with everything in their world, including their physical comfort, level of knowledge, emotional state, quality of sensory input, and spiritual welfare, we have to recognize that they need to communicate to make changes that will resolve the dissonances between the way things are and how they might be.[13]

Breaking through the degree–kind barrier

People living with a dementia may well withdraw from communication, but it doesn't mean they have no desire to communicate, or that they cannot be reached. A striking example is the film of Naomi Feil's interaction with Gladys Wilson,[14] which many people have found remarkable and heartening. Gladys appears completely unable to communicate. Feil begins talking to her, touching her face and singing to her. Over the course of several minutes, we see Gladys start to respond, first by using her hand to rhythmically follow the beat of the song, then by filling in gaps in the chorus. Finally, she's able to answer simple questions. The first time I showed the film to some students, I saw their eyes open wide with surprise and joy

---

13   Wray (2020b, p. 250)
14   Feil (2009)

in seeing these responses from someone whom they had, almost certainly, categorized as unable to communicate – different in *kind*. Now, they saw that inside this person with advanced dementia there was still something they could recognize as being like them. Gladys Wilson remained, in some regard, different only in *degree*.

To help avoid people being categorized as only ever different in kind – or indeed only ever different in degree – I've drawn up the Manifesto for Caring Care (Figure 7.2).[15] The aim of this manifesto is to offer basic principles for orienting towards, and back towards, *different in degree* wherever possible, without denying the value of *different in kind* in certain circumstances. It invites us to be flexible and alert, and to regularly challenge our assumptions.

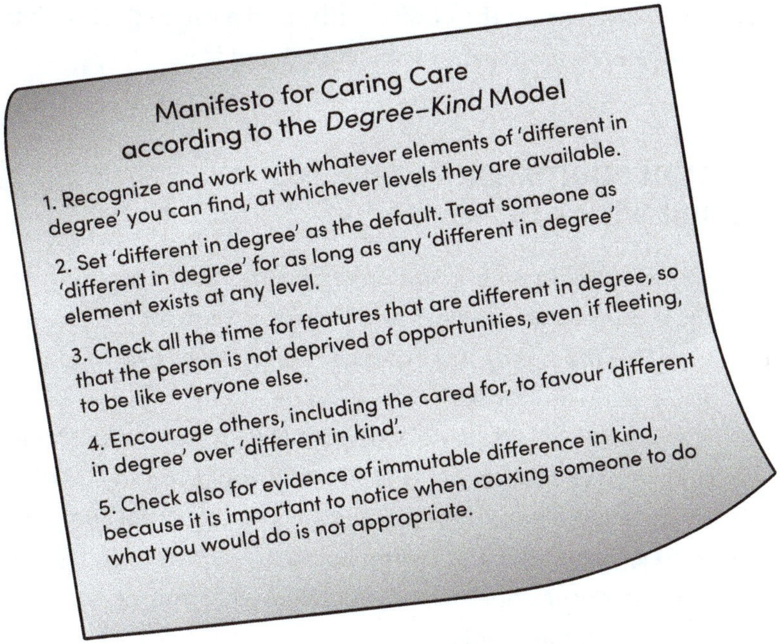

> **Manifesto for Caring Care according to the *Degree–Kind* Model**
>
> 1. Recognize and work with whatever elements of 'different in degree' you can find, at whichever levels they are available.
>
> 2. Set 'different in degree' as the default. Treat someone as 'different in degree' for as long as any 'different in degree' element exists at any level.
>
> 3. Check all the time for features that are different in degree, so that the person is not deprived of opportunities, even if fleeting, to be like everyone else.
>
> 4. Encourage others, including the cared for, to favour 'different in degree' over 'different in kind'.
>
> 5. Check also for evidence of immutable difference in kind, because it is important to notice when coaxing someone to do what you would do is not appropriate.

Figure 7.2: Manifesto for Caring Care

Overall, the best way to avoid Kitwood's malignant social psychology is to treat people living with a dementia, where possible, as having some similarity to ourselves. This is how we can maximize their

---

15   Adapted from Wray (2020b, p. 243)

chance of feeling connected and valued. According to item 2 in the manifesto, we will use the continuums for different functions to find any possible opportunities to treat the person as *different in degree*. Item 5, however, reminds us to remain aware that sometimes the *degree* perspective could put too much pressure on them and be difficult or distressing.

Although this manifesto may increase the emotional stress on the family member or carer, who might find it easier to dismiss the person's actions as 'abnormal', there are two things that should encourage us to apply it. The first is that the manifesto raises our awareness of what's going on, which is better than simply making assumptions without thought. The second is that a tension between the advantages and disadvantages of *degree* and *kind* is inevitable. There's no way to make the choice without having to deal with that tension, so there's no reason to shy away from it.

ACTION POINTS FOR PEOPLE LIVING WITH A DEMENTIA

1. Write letters to your loved ones and friends, reassuring them that you care about them and thanking them for their love and care. Tell them that you'll always feel this way, even if, one day, you can no longer say so.
2. If someone asked you about your life, preferences, interests and what you most care about, what would you say? Write this information down. Then you know it's available for someone to read if, in the future, you aren't able to tell them. You may even find the description useful yourself if you struggle sometimes to recall all the details.
3. Think about all the different aspects of yourself: your abilities, your history, your relationships, your feelings, your physical capabilities, your senses. Humans are so complicated, but it's our choice what we focus on most. Be aware of, and glad of, those aspects of yourself that dementia isn't changing, because they enable you to continue being the same person that you

always were. If you write your thoughts down, you could share them with your family to help them support you in bringing out these aspects.

ACTION POINTS FOR FAMILIES, FRIENDS AND PROFESSIONALS

1. Reassure the person living with the dementia that even if some aspects of their abilities and knowledge have changed, you're still most interested in the core features of who they are, which won't change.

2. Write a card to the person living with a dementia, expressing your love and appreciation of them and/or recalling some funny or enjoyable event. Ask other family members and friends to do the same. Such messages can become treasured possessions that remind the person that they're loved, even if they're no longer sure who wrote them.

3. Similarly, help them make a record of their life, because reminiscences can connect them to their core identity.

4. Thinking about the person living with a dementia whom you know, make your own version of Figure 7.1, where you identify where on the continuum they are for each function. Add extra functions if you wish. You could also write down some examples of what's different only in *degree* and what you feel is different in *kind*.

5. For any features that are different in kind for a person living with a dementia whom you know, think about whether or not it benefits them when you view them in this way (either answer is possible). Now consider what's more beneficial for you. If different in degree is better for them and different in kind is better for you (or vice versa), how could you proceed, so you accommodate the needs of both of you?

6. Think about how you might apply the manifesto in Figure 7.2 in your daily life. What issues might arise and how would you deal with them?

ACTION POINTS FOR BYSTANDERS

1. Only engaging occasionally with people living with a dementia can mean it's easy to view them as different in kind, since they're a greater contrast to most people in our daily experience. Think about people living with a dementia whom you sometimes encounter. Do you think you tend to view them as *different in degree* or *different in kind*? Imagine viewing them in the opposite way. How might that lead you to behave towards them? What advantages and disadvantages could there be to changing your view?

2. Write down all the words that come to mind when you think of someone living with a dementia. Then sort the words into three sets: positive, negative and neutral. Look at the relative size of those sets and consider what any differences signify. If the negative set is largest, what could you do to alter how you think about people living with a dementia that might change the balance if you did this exercise again in the future?[16]

3. If you observe family and professional carers engaging in malignant social psychology, what could you do to steer them back towards a more humane approach? What support might they need?

---

16   My thanks to Maria Nicol for suggesting this exercise.

CHAPTER EIGHT

Dementia and Deception

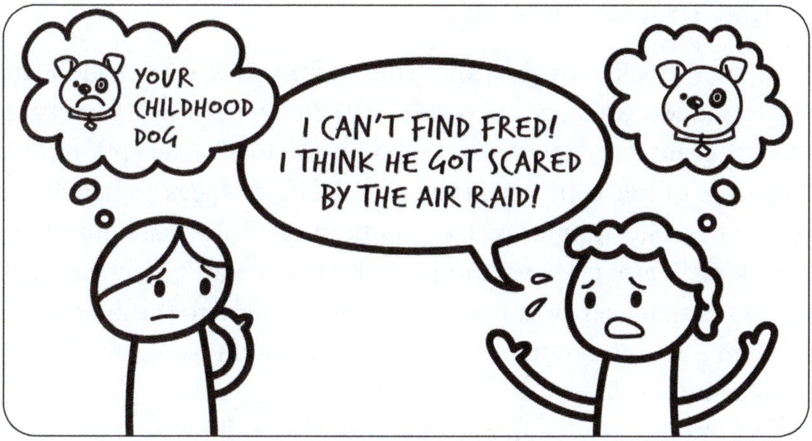

Elsie Mill

At the beginning of his book *Tell Mrs Mill Her Husband Is Still Dead*, David Clegg recounts the following scene:

> Every day at four o'clock Elsie Mill, slowly and with great effort, made her way to the locked door of the residential unit and waited to be let out. She said her husband, who everyone but Elsie knew had died twenty years before, was due back from work and that he would be expecting his tea. ... One day a nurse told me how they prevented her obstructing the entrance. Once Elsie was in position one of the staff would call from the office saying that her sister was on the phone. Using her two sticks Elsie would then take ten minutes to walk the length of the short corridor, which was enough time to tell

her that her sister had hung up. She would then walk slowly back to the door. Ten minutes later they would do it again. Repeatedly tricking a frail old woman and then hoping she would forget seemed so contrary to care, so mocking and so wrong that the next time I found her at the door I told her the truth. I said she must have loved her husband very much since he had passed away years before and that if she wanted to we could go to her room and look through her photographs and she could tell me about him. At first she said I was mistaken and that I was confusing her with someone else. Then, as I gently repeated what I had said, she visibly relaxed and said I was right, 'Then he's not outside, is he?'[1]

Clegg was shocked by the callousness of the staff who made Elsie Mill repeatedly walk up the corridor with hope in her heart and back down it again with a sense of disappointment. The deception took advantage of her vulnerabilities – her desire to speak to her sister, her poor recollection for recent events and her physical limitations in walking. It also gave more importance to the staff's practical challenge of keeping her away from the front door than to the underlying problem – her yearning to be needed and useful to someone who cared about her.

Although that was an extreme example, telling lies to people living with a dementia is far from unusual. Family and professional carers often feel that telling the whole truth would be unwise or undesirable. Even with Elsie Mill, we can imagine the staff being at their wits' end, trying to prevent her slipping out of the building and wandering off. It's certainly a pity they couldn't think of a more dignified solution, but let's just consider what other choices they had.

They could have told her the truth – that her husband was dead. Since she had a poor memory, they'd have had to do it many times a day. Unless the staff were as gentle in breaking the news as Clegg was and had time to support her through hearing this bad news (as if for the first time), they could well have left her in a constant state of distress about the bereavement.

---

1   Clegg (2010, p. 11)

Alternatively, they could have distracted her in a less cruel way – by getting her into a room with an activity going on, say. But how could they persuade her to abandon her responsibility for getting home to make her husband's tea? They'd need to explain why she didn't need to worry – perhaps *He phoned and said he'd be late home* (lie), *He's coming to see you this evening* (lie), *You don't have to go home yet, and I'll tell you when it's time* (lie), or *He's already had his tea* (lie). Even something like *It's okay, you don't have to worry about your husband, I promise* would still be, at the very least, misleading, given what Elsie believed.

In one research study, 71 per cent of medical doctors said that they had lied to a person living with a dementia at some point.[2] In another study, which included nurses, unqualified care staff and occupational therapists as well as doctors, the figure was 96.4 per cent.[3] Studies like these have also revealed that some topics are more likely to be lied about than others. One ward sister said staff would 'lie through their teeth' to get a person living with a dementia to take medication, but that it was contrary to professional ethics to be untruthful when discussing diagnosis or end-of-life care.[4]

Deception comes up as an option when the person we're communicating with has different beliefs about the world from us. As we saw in Chapters 4 and 5, communication only works if there's some overlap between what the speaker and listener each know. If that overlap isn't there, then one person is going to have to take on some of the beliefs of the other. It's just a question of who.

When a person living with a dementia is told the truth about something they don't know, or that they believe is different from how it is, then their knowledge is being shifted so it overlaps with what the speaker knows or believes. They have to fit that new information into their existing knowledge and beliefs. Elsie Mill didn't know her husband was dead. If someone told her the truth, she'd have to cope with the consequences of that new knowledge – whether surprise, distress or confusion. Since she wouldn't retain the information for

---

2   Caiazza et al. (2016)
3   James et al. (2006)
4   Turner et al. (2016, p. 865)

long, telling the truth to her would have two major downsides. She'd experience the strong emotions associated with the new information, yet it wouldn't solve the problem in the long run.

For these reasons, it's often judged better for the *other* person to shift ground. That means setting aside their own knowledge and beliefs about the situation, and 'buying into' what the person living with the dementia believes. This is what Sue did in Chapter 6. Her husband Trevor believed he was still working as a policeman. Instead of insisting he alter his beliefs to match hers, she gave him the impression that she also believed he was still a policeman. With that overlap of beliefs, they could communicate satisfactorily – she could ensure he felt calm and content by reassuring him that she'd take care of the police paperwork.

However, saying and implying things that one knows to be untrue goes against the grain for most people, and deceiving others is generally viewed as disrespectful, even morally wrong. As a result, families and professional carers often experience guilt or anxiety about deceiving people living with a dementia. Given such concerns, why is deception used so much? And what exactly counts as a lie? Are some types of lie worse than others? These are some of the questions we explore in this chapter.

What counts as lying?
Direct and indirect lies
Suppose a person living with a dementia says that she wants to use the car to go somewhere, but in fact it's no longer safe for her to drive. Her stressed son wants to avoid a long argument about whether she should or shouldn't drive. It's much easier to say that the key's missing, or that the car's broken down. However, it's a blatant lie, likely to make the liar feel uneasy and guilty. As a result, indirect types of deception are commonly used instead. For instance, the son might disconnect a wire in the car. Now he can honestly say that the car won't start. Or he gives the key to the next-door neighbour, and now he can say, *Oh, Mary's got the key at the moment.* Are these lies? It depends on how exact we want to be about the meaning of the

word 'lie' but the person living with the dementia is certainly being misled.[5] Yet the son can argue that he didn't actually say anything untrue.

As that example shows, it's possible to be both truthful and un-truthful at the same time. Consider what my mother said when my siblings and I asked her whether Father Christmas really existed: 'For as long as there are little children, there'll always be a Father Christmas.' Well, that's true. It's just that she knew we'd interpret it in a particular way that preserved a falsehood she'd already told us. She knew we didn't have the ability yet to read between the lines and infer information that wasn't actually stated directly.

To see through our mother's statement, we'd have needed to do something that's cognitively rather complicated – map out how the world would look from her point of view if there actually was no Father Christmas and she was trying to prevent us realizing that. Only then would her statement be transparent to us. Aged seven or eight, we couldn't do all that mental gymnastics. In fact, to us the statement was reassurance that Father Christmas did exist, since it was clearly true that there will always be little children. In contrast to our poor map of *her* knowledge, our mother had a clear map of what *our* existing knowledge was, and where it did and didn't overlap with her own. That enabled her to steer a course within the bounds of the truth, without actually bursting the bubble of our magical false belief.

It's not only children that we lie to indirectly – it's other adults as well. For instance, if my friend asks me if I like her new coat and I think it's hideous, what am I going to say? I might say, truthfully, *I really like the belt.* I haven't said I hate the coat, which would upset her. I haven't said I like it, which would be a lie. But I have sort of lied, in the sense that I said something positive about her coat even though my views were negative. Here's a particularly clever example, created by Ronald Posner.[6]

---

5   For a discussion of the meanings of terms and the nuances of deception, see Wray (2020b, p. 220ff).
6   Posner (1980, p. 179)

The first mate of a ship is often drunk, and the captain gets fed up. He wants the first mate to get into trouble when they get back to port. So he writes in the log, *Today, March 23rd, the first mate was drunk*. The first mate is angry, and wants to get his own back, but he knows he mustn't lie in the log book. So, he writes, *Today, March 26th, the captain was not drunk*.

It's a true statement – the captain was, indeed, not drunk. However, the first mate knows that anyone reading that entry will wonder why this fact was worth noting down and will assume that not being drunk was an exception to the usual pattern. In short, the mate puts an untrue idea into the reader's head, even though he hasn't actually written anything untrue himself.

This sort of mind game is possible because of how listeners use the context to extract meaning from what they hear. They want to know why something was said and why in that way (as outlined in Chapters 4 and 5). Crafty speakers or writers can anticipate what listeners or readers are bringing to that interpretation and exploit it.

People living with a dementia are particularly vulnerable to indirect lying for several reasons. First, dementia makes cognitive processing more difficult, so it's harder for them to keep up with complicated ideas and see through mind games. Second, they may not be able to take in, recall and track all the relevant context, such as what happened last time, why the speaker might say what they've said or why the claim is implausible. Third, if they have their own beliefs about the context (e.g. that they're 18 years old rather than 86), they'll begin with certain assumptions when they try to make sense of what's said to them – and the speaker may well exploit that fact. Fourth, people living with a dementia are generally very reliant on those around them and have to trust in others' goodwill and honesty. If the person they're relying on for getting a desired change in their world tells them that what they want isn't possible, there may be little they can do about it.

False environments

I mentioned in Chapter 5 the Dutch dementia care village called Hogeweyk.[7] It's been praised as a particularly supportive and caring environment to live in, and there's been interest in developing similar villages elsewhere.[8] Yet its entire basis is deception, in that it appears to be an ordinary village.[9] The medical and care staff are disguised as regular inhabitants[10] and most residents don't realize that it's a dementia care facility. The extreme level of pretence has been likened to the movie *The Truman Show*, in which the main character in a soap opera is born and lives entirely on the film set, believing it's real life.[11] As with the film set in *The Truman Show*, at Hogeweyk a great deal of trouble has been taken to create the illusion of a real village.

Even though Hogeweyk remains unusual as a deceptive environment, more limited versions are encountered quite often. Many residential care homes decorate a corridor to look like a street (Figure 8.1) or paint images onto walls that appear to give perspective and distance. Sometimes bus stops are painted on walls, a small coffee area is presented as a regular café (Figure 8.2) or rooms are filled with the décor and objects of several decades ago. The intention is to provide familiarity in a world that's otherwise potentially over-clinical and bewildering – and presumably it works. However, there's also an argument that this sort of misrepresentation is confusing in its own right.[12] For example, one researcher describes what happened at a dementia day care centre that had been decorated to look like a commercial restaurant: 'People with [Alzheimer's disease]…often acted as if they were at a coffee shop and were confused when they could not order what they wanted and were not able to leave at will.'[13]

---

7   https://hogeweyk.dementiavillage.com
8   Gallagher (2018)
9   Moisse (2012)
10 Sampson (2014)
11 Planos (2014)
12 That is the argument, for example, of reality orientation (e.g. Bowlby 1991; O'Connell et al. 2007) and cognitive stimulation therapy (e.g. Comas-Herrera and Knapp 2016). It is also the position taken in the enquiry into the use of deception in dementia care by Kirtley and Williamson (2016).
13 Guendouzi and Savage (2017, p. 332)

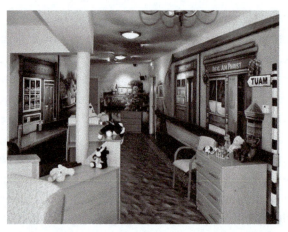

Figure 8.1: A corridor decorated as a street[14]

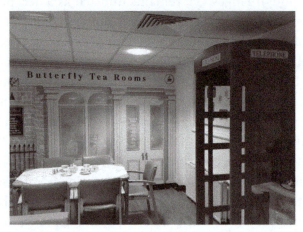

Figure 8.2: A wall decorated like a café frontage[15]

Another type of deception is intended to prevent people living with a dementia from straying outside certain areas of the premises. Doors might be disguised, painted in an unattractive way or fitted with mirrors so the person believes someone's walking towards them and turns away.[16] A black mat in front of a door might be used as a barrier, since people living with a dementia easily mistake dark mats

---

14 Reproduced with the permission of Central Park Nursing Home, Clonberne, Ballinasloe, Co. Galway, Ireland.

15 Reproduced with the permission of Airedale NHS Foundation Trust, Keighley, West Yorkshire, UK.

16 Namazi, Rosner and Calkins (1989)

for holes in the ground.[17] Again, we can see the reasons for taking such measures. It's more practical and arguably more caring to create a barrier than constantly have to tell people living with a dementia that they can't go through that door or into that area. But some would view this sort of deception as particularly unacceptable since it directly exploits the disabilities in cognitive and visual processing that dementia causes.

'Going along with'

In many approaches to dementia care, it's claimed that staff never lie but that they will 'go along with' what the person says and not contradict them. For example, if the person claims that they have to get up and go to work, they won't be told they're wrong, but rather helped to dress appropriately and have a suitably hearty breakfast for the day ahead. (By then, it's hoped, the person will no longer recall their mission and will settle down to some activity on the premises.) The rationale for this method is clear – why get into persistent contradiction with someone if they can experience energy and purpose by operating within their own beliefs? Sometimes, there's even proactive support for the false belief, such as giving the person activities that imply they are still working in their old job.[18] Recall how Sue supported her husband Trevor's belief that he was still working in the police station by agreeing to do his paperwork for him.

For those who feel that even 'going along with' is unacceptable, the person's beliefs might instead be used as the springboard for a conversation that doesn't involve any deception. For example, if a person living with a dementia speaks of her father being at home waiting for her, a carer might get her to talk about her father. This could help with understanding why she's connecting with memories of him – perhaps she feels abandoned or needs reassurance.

However, even here there can be difficulties, because of the way language works. Suppose the person says, *I'm looking for my father*, and the carer says, *What does he look like?* The use of the present

17   Klosterman (2014)
18   Dementia Care Matters (2016)

tense implies agreement that he's alive. Yet using the past tense, *What did he look like?*, would signal the bad news that he's dead.[19] This is a quandary that is difficult to avoid – in effect the language can sometimes force a choice between a deceptive statement and a difficult truth.

Are some types of lie worse than others?

Most people would feel that *I'm sure Snowy didn't suffer when she got run over* is a 'better' lie than *No, I didn't take the money out of your purse.* There are various reasons why some lies seem more acceptable than others, including who benefits from the lie, and what the consequences are if the liar gets found out. We often use the expression 'white lie' for deceptions that we consider harmless; and on a similar basis, deceiving people living with a dementia is often referred to as 'therapeutic lying', that is, lying that's intended to improve, rather than damage, the person's wellbeing.

Who benefits from the deception?

Let's first unpack the question of who benefits from a lie. Sometimes, it's clear that all the benefit comes to the deceiver. Imagine a person living with a dementia has a professional carer who comes to his house each day to help him with important daily tasks. Today, he asks the carer to take him out into the garden. But the carer doesn't want to do that because the mud will ruin her shoes. So, she tells him the door's locked and (untruthfully) that she doesn't know where the key is. This is a lie that advantages the carer and disadvantages the client.

But often, things won't be as clear cut. Suppose the reason the carer isn't keen to take the client into the garden is because she only has half an hour to complete a set of tasks, including making his lunch and ensuring he's clean and comfortable. She might also be concerned about him falling. He might not appreciate these issues and so not understand why going into the garden is a problem. She

---

19   McElveen (2015)

might feel that it's not a good idea to get into a long explanation, so it's easier all round if she just tells him that going outside isn't possible. She's still lying to him, but now, although it's still for her benefit in various respects, it's also for his.

Given the massive risk to people living with a dementia of losing their basic freedoms and rights, it's important to take seriously the possibility that other people's preferences get prioritized too easily. Yet we can't ignore the needs and concerns of those in positions of responsibility, who can find their caring role very stressful. People living with a dementia can't always make a full and balanced judgement about a situation, so might have expectations that are unreasonable or impractical. For instance, they might not appreciate their own limitations, or might believe they're in a different situation from the one they're actually in, or think they have responsibilities to fulfil that they don't actually have, such as caring for their children or getting home to their parents.

One common context where lying is regarded as beneficial to people living with a dementia is when it protects them from emotional distress. Here we need to separate out two situations – when something distressing has just happened and the person has not been told, and when it's happened previously and the person no longer recalls the information. Regarding new information, in their detailed report on the ethics of lying to people living with a dementia, Kirtley and Williamson argue that it's not good for a person's wellbeing to shield them from the bad news. 'Stress and distress are part of being human', so 'one must also allow them to experience the full range of adult emotions including doubt, uncertainty, sadness and change'.[20] According to this view, a person living with a dementia should be informed when their spouse passes away, even though the news will be painful. There are practical reasons too, of course, since the spouse will now not visit any more, and because it might be felt appropriate for the person living with the dementia to attend the funeral.

However, when the person has been told this news before and no longer recalls it, a different approach is often taken. Rather than

---

20   Kirtley and Williamson (2016, p. 23)

rerun the breaking of the news, evasion or deception is often used. The argument is that each time the news is broken, it's as if for the first time, leading to another experience of shock and distress, which is unkind and unnecessary. This is an entirely reasonable argument on the surface, but when we dig a little deeper, we see why problems can arise.

The decision not to tell the truth relies on the person living with the dementia having no recollection of the information at all. But we should be wary of assuming that recall is all or nothing. It could be that, based on what they were told previously, they still half-know. They might suspect their loved one has died, but not be able to recall enough detail to be sure. So, they might ask where the person is. If they're now told he's gone for a walk, and next time they're told he's upstairs, then that will be difficult to reconcile with their niggling belief that he's died, leaving them confused and unsure what to feel.

If that's an argument for sticking to the truth, here's one for not doing so. As discussed later in this chapter, the emotional after-effect of hearing bad news could last beyond the person's recall of what the news was. If they're told bad news repeatedly, these negative feelings could build up into a huge emotional burden that they can't explain or reason away.

What this indicates is that no caring family member or professional is likely to be certain how to proceed on a given occasion, because there's no single right thing to do. It'll depend on their best guess about how the person will respond. Anticipating my discussion of the SPECAL approach, below, here's an example of how the truth about some sad news was broken to someone by lying to them, because this was viewed as the kindest approach to take.

Jack, living with a dementia, didn't know that Richard, one of the staff at his support group, had died.[21] The staff were concerned about upsetting Jack with this news, but they still felt he ought to be told. They used the fact that both Jack and Richard had spent time in the army to say, 'Isn't it a pity about poor old Richard? But at least he got

---

21   This story was recounted to me by Zoë Elkins, and it took place in the context of the SPECAL method that's described later in this chapter.

a five-gun salute.' Jack apparently expressed surprise, then saluted Richard and had no negative reaction.

What they'd done was present this new information as if Jack had been told it before. By doing this, they created a situation in which Jack would be less likely to react as if he were hearing the news for the first time, even though he was. In other words, they used two interacting features of Jack's present cognitive capabilities: that he had poor recall for previous events, and that he *knew* he did. They led him to assume that he'd heard the news before and not retained it. The way Jack was treated here is multi-layered. We need to recognize that the underlying purpose was to tell him the truth about Richard's death. To do so, some measure of deception was used, in presenting the information as old news. They exploited his cognitive vulnerabilities but did so in order to minimize his distress. So, was this an acceptable use of deception, given that it was done for his benefit *and* that he ended up knowing the truth?

Getting away with it

One of the major risks of lying is getting found out, though it's up for debate whether it's more acceptable to lie if you think you'll get away with it or if you think you're leaving the other person a reasonable chance of finding you out. So, what makes some lies easier to detect than others? There's a good reason why we refer to *the* truth but *a* lie – there are many different ways to lie. Since one lie easily creates the need for another, and another, it's common to end up with a whole web of deception that's difficult to keep track of. Once you start a deception, you have to see it through. Having helped someone dress smartly because they believe they have to go to work, what are you going to do if they're now standing at the door with the briefcase you gave them, wanting to go and catch the bus?

We saw earlier how people at a day centre decorated to look like a commercial restaurant got confused when they couldn't order what they wanted and leave when they chose. That was a deception not followed through. And at the Hogeweyk village, huge effort is needed to sustain the pretence that it's a normal village community in the face of various inevitable contrary indications, such as not being able to leave the grounds, or people saying things that don't quite ring true.

Overall, it is likely to be easier to get away with a lie when *speaking* to a person living with a dementia, though the situation may be more complicated than it seems. Deceivers rely heavily on people living with a dementia not seeing through their lies or, if they do, not being able to piece together how they've been deceived. However, as we saw earlier, knowledge is not necessarily all or nothing, and deceptions may strike the person as odd and unlikely, even if they can't put their finger on why. Meanwhile, if a person living with a dementia challenges a lie, they are at risk of power games, as the other person simply out-argues them, insisting that the lie is actually the truth. Only if family and carers are willing to back down with an apology for having made a mistake can the person feel vindicated and secure in their capacity to judge a situation, rather than being overwhelmed by false counterarguments.

There are certain instances of deception that seem particularly likely to be detected, even by a person living with a dementia. One is Simulated Presence, or SimPres, a therapeutic approach intended to help calm people living with a dementia by giving them access to the voice of a family member. The family member is recorded talking about events in the person's life associated with positive emotions. The recording is set up as one side of a phone conversation with pauses for the person to respond. The recording can be used repeatedly: '...it is perceived by the individual to represent a fresh, live telephone call each time it is used, because the person with [Alzheimer's] cannot recall that the tape has been played before'.[22] As it turns out, research on SimPres has only low levels of scientific reliability and is inconclusive regarding effectiveness,[23] so we don't know with any certainty if individuals can even benefit from it. And two underlying assumptions are concerning: that even a badly impaired memory can't still surface that sense of *déjà vu* about exactly repeated events, which were sometimes as often as twice daily; and that a person

22   Camberg et al. (1999, p. 447)
23   Abraha et al. (2020)

wouldn't notice the unresponsiveness of the recorded speaker to what they said in reply. Of course, one assumes that SimPres would only be used with those who were considered likely to be taken in by it, but since the cognitive abilities of people living with a dementia can vary considerably from day to day, care would still be needed.

In sum, deceiving people living with a dementia is far from straightforward, and it may create as many problems as it solves. The approach described next brings the pros and cons of continual deception into particular focus.

The case of 'SPECAL' – Contented Dementia

One method for interacting with people living with dementia is worth special discussion. It's called SPECAL (Specialized Early Care for Alzheimer's) but is more commonly known as Contented Dementia, because of Oliver James's[24] successful book of that name. There are two characteristics about SPECAL that mark it out. One is how positively it is viewed by those who have adopted it. The other is that the UK Alzheimer's Society singled it out for criticism, because of its systematic approach to deception.[25] SPECAL helps us draw out the conflict between benefits and rights when it comes to deceiving people living with a dementia. A full description of SPECAL would take too much space here, so I'll just summarize the aspects of it that are most relevant to the question of deception.[26]

The basic priority in SPECAL is to minimize the amount of anxiety and distress that people living with a dementia undergo. When something slightly disturbing, annoying or worrying happens to someone without a dementia, they can work it through in their mind till it makes sense to them and they can handle its effects. For instance, imagine I was on the street and someone pushed past me, knocking me over, so I fell and hurt my leg. Later, I could recall the events, think about the fact that I felt angry with the person who pushed me, consider whether they did it on purpose, run back

---

24 James (2008)
25 Alzheimer's Society (2020)
26 For fuller descriptions, see James (2008) and Wray (2020b, pp. 229–237).

through the apology they gave me and how they helped me up, and link the current pain in my leg to these events.

However, if that accident happened to someone living with Alzheimer's, they might not be able to recall what happened. All they'd know is that their leg hurt for some reason and that they had the negative feelings associated with having felt anger. They'd no longer know what they were angry about. They'd be stuck with their feelings and have no explanation for them. It could be very frightening for them to discover an injury and strong negative emotion that seemed to have just come out of nowhere.

According to SPECAL, when people living with a dementia are in this sort of situation, they look for an explanation for their experience. If they have poor access to recent events in memory, they're likely to search their more reliable older memories. As a result, they might come to believe that their leg hurts because of, say, a car accident they had many years ago, caused by a schoolmate who often made them angry. Obviously, if they start talking about what they believe happened, it's going to confuse those around them, who might not even know about that car accident and schoolmate, so nothing will make any sense. As a result, the person living with the dementia may find that the other person challenges what they're saying, which could then annoy and frustrate them.

Confusion, frustration and annoyance are natural responses for most people if they discover that communication has broken down. But while the unimpaired person in the conversation can go off and think about what was said, and perhaps work out what went wrong, the person living with the dementia may soon no longer even recall the conversation, and only have a persistent feeling that something unpleasant happened. To explain the feeling, they may go once again into the more distant past, looking for a reliable memory that matches the feeling. Now they're drawing on *another* memory that the other person won't recognize, which will cause more confusion and negative reactions. In this way, these traumatic experiences can build and build, till the person living with the dementia is in a state of agitation that is difficult to quell.

The SPECAL approach aims to turn things round, by helping

people living with a dementia link instead to enjoyable, comforting experiences from the past. This is achieved in two ways. First, everything is done to avoid any negative experiences in the present, so the person doesn't need to look for matching negative experiences in the past. Second, steps are taken to help the person access the most comfortable and safe time in their life, by saying things that chime with it. Both tactics focus on helping the person living with the dementia feel content and safe, and this is why those who adopt the approach like it so much. They report that their loved ones are 'more at peace with themselves', more social and more communicative, and have greater self-esteem[27] – all of these attributes are indications of greater emotional reserve (see Chapter 2).

The issue, however, is that in order to create that safe space, a false world has to be created and sustained. To avoid negative experiences in the present, it may be necessary in SPECAL to withhold information about what's happening, or lie about it. In some instances, people will conspire to create complicated lies about a situation, intended to let the person feel comfortable or valued. For instance, one person who liked playing bridge but struggled to recall the rules was taken to bridge sessions where everyone else agreed to pretend that they were playing normally when in fact they were making all sorts of allowances.[28] In another case, a person living with a dementia was 'tricked' into attending a support group meeting by being told he'd been invited to give advice to the group.[29] A woman who had been good at sewing arrived at the same group to find it set up as a sewing group in which she could be the 'expert'.[30]

This sort of intricate deception is extended to the second aspect of SPECAL. Over a long period of time, the person living with the dementia is observed, so as to note which specific information is most likely to deceive them successfully. For instance, if someone close to them isn't in the room, what sort of explanation about their absence will most reliably keep them calm? Typically, it'll be an explanation

---

27   Pritchard and Dewing (1999, pp. 7: 8,17)
28   James (2008, pp. 32–40)
29   Pritchard and Dewing (1999, p. 7: 4)
30   Godel (2000, p. 21)

that resonates with a happy period in the past, when they weren't anxious about that person not being present for a while. That explanation is then used, even though it's not true. For example, one daughter who used this approach with her father when her mother was out of the house said:

> This worked brilliantly with Dad. Whenever he asked where Mum was, he was incredibly happy with her *being at the club* and we could have a positive conversation which settled him, and he asked less and less where Mum was. We used it for seven years, even when Dad was in the rest-home.[31]

It seems that he was satisfied believing his wife was out doing what she'd always done. It's reasoned in SPECAL that a small number of explanations can be used repeatedly, since the person won't recall having been told them before. The net effect is that the person is sustained in a permanent state of contentment, with no negative emotions.[32]

So, which is better? Telling the truth and risking people living with a dementia feeling perpetually anxious and agitated, or wrapping them up in fabrications that keep them feeling contented? Which way an individual jumps must depend substantially on how squeamish they are about creating and sustaining a web of lies. The Alzheimer's Society maintains that it's unethical to be deliberately and repeatedly untruthful to people who are so vulnerable to others' deceit.[33] SPECAL supporters would no doubt argue that provided the purpose of the deception is to build and preserve contentment, it's better for the unimpaired person to deal with a bit of unease than leave the person living with the dementia with negative feelings.

Another type of criticism against SPECAL comes in the in-depth report on truth and deception in dementia by Kirtley and Williamson. It questions whether SPECAL makes accurate assumptions about how dementia affects people's ability to reason and retain

---

31   Maria Nicol, personal communication
32   James (2008)
33   Alzheimer's Society (2020)

information.[34] And certainly the SPECAL approach isn't suitable for anyone with sufficient memory capacity to notice the repetition or to question the truth of what's said to them. Furthermore, to get all the information into place, the SPECAL process needs to begin early on, and during that period the person living with the dementia is being observed for how they react to different things and also what they tend to say, without being told that this is happening.

For these various reasons, there are certainly grounds for being unsure if SPECAL is an ethically acceptable approach. Given its appeal to its users, however, it would be useful to see its effectiveness evaluated in some formal scientific studies.

What do people living with a dementia think about being lied to?

It appears that people living with a dementia are rarely asked what they think about the idea of being lied to. It's obviously a sensitive topic, but as diagnoses are made earlier and earlier, it's becoming more possible to allow people with a diagnosis to express their views. Different aspects need to be separated out here – what it feels like to be told a difficult truth, and what it feels like to be told a plausible lie.

One person living with a dementia who contributed to Kirtley and Williamson's report on deception recognized that she sometimes didn't want to accept the truth: 'I become convinced that I am right in the face of explanations which attempt to prove to me that I am wrong. I resent and resist these attempts and experience them as oppressive.'[35] Even where people living with a dementia recognize that their disease can cause them to have false beliefs, giving up those beliefs may be difficult because it's linked to giving up self-determination and self-belief (see Chapter 4). The same person quoted above also said, 'My caregivers, family and friends frequently assume they know when I am confused. They think they know what I am thinking. I get angry about this.'[36]

---

34 Williamson and Kirtley (2016, pp. 46–47)
35 Williamson and Kirtley (2016, p. 38)
36 Williamson and Kirtley (2016, p. 38)

The situation seems almost impossible. On the one hand, if the unimpaired person's truth is always insisted on, the person living with the dementia will feel powerless, not listened to and, often, confused. On the other hand, if the unimpaired person simply agrees with whatever the person living with the dementia says, that could be seen as patronizing. And it might not work all that well, since there's no guarantee that a person's dementia will deliver a consistent alternative set of truths. If it doesn't, then both parties will end up confused.

When it comes to be lied to, understandably people living with a dementia are concerned about their rights and dignity. But, interestingly, when researchers gave 14 people living with Alzheimer's a set of scenarios in which a lie might be told, the response was mixed.[37] The scenarios were:

1. A gentleman with dementia asks for his 'deceased' dog. The carer tells him his dog is asleep in the laundry room or is out for a walk. When the gentleman is told his dog is dead, he gets distressed.

2. A carer does not correct a resident who asks to go home to see a deceased relative.

3. A lady with dementia urgently needs chiropody but refuses to see the chiropodist. A carer tells the lady that she had already agreed to see the chiropodist, when in fact she has not.

4. A carer hides the car keys of a gentleman so he cannot drive.

5. A carer tells a lady that her daughter is coming to visit when in fact she is not. This is done in order to get the lady out of bed.

6. Mirrors are placed on exit doors as a distraction in order to stop people 'wandering'.

The participants in this study (who were living with Alzheimer's) considered it demeaning to be lied to and were concerned at how it could reduce their personal freedom. They were concerned that if

---

37   Day et al. (2011)

people living with a dementia found out they'd been lied to it would undermine their trust in others in future. Therefore, they felt that lying was less of a problem if the person being lied to was unlikely to see through the deception.[38] It was also reasonable to lie if it would protect the person from physical or emotional harm. In their view, being lied to by a close friend or a relative was worse than being lied to by a professional carer. Finally, they felt that any kind of deception should be decided on case-by-case, so that there was no practice of habitual lying.

This last point is significant, considering how SPECAL and several other approaches to communication – including the Hogeweyk dementia village – set up and sustain a false world. Of course, each individual will have their own view on whether it's acceptable to be subjected to systematic, pre-planned deception if it's for their own good.[39] Jennifer Bute, a person living with Alzheimer's who has made it her mission to improve our understanding of what the experience is like, is comfortable with it:

> Rather than make a 'scene' of having to go, say 'I am just going to the loo' or '[I] need to make a drink' so that I am happy to 'let you go'. I might then forget you haven't returned but still feel happy rather than feel disturbed because something is not right by your departure.[40]

But others will no doubt feel that when they are lied to in this way, it removes the link with reality that dementia gradually undermines.

Does lying mean we're treating people as different in kind?

Finally, let's link the discussion in this chapter with that of Chapter 7. We saw there how people living with a dementia can get treated either as fundamentally different in *kind* – not like everyone else and

---

38 Day et al. (2011, p. 825)
39 For a discussion of the relationship between premeditated deception, individualized deception and flexibility in the use of deception, see Wray (2020b, pp. 234–236).
40 Bute (2010)

not like their former self – or as different in *degree* – experiencing the same things as everyone else, just in a more extreme way. When we view someone as different in kind it increases the risk of treating them with contempt. The question is, does lying to a person living with a dementia mean we're treating them as different in kind?

At first glance, deceiving people living with a dementia seems to indicate that they're being treated as different in kind, because the general social rule is to be honest. But in fact, as we've seen already, well-meant deception is rife in society. We tell children lies to protect them from uncomfortable information (or to help them sustain a fantasy world), and we lie to our friends because it's more kind-hearted. So, can we really say that people living with a dementia are being treated any differently if we lie to them? Could it be argued that we'd be treating them differently from everyone else if we *refused* to lie to them, even when was more humane to do so?

Individuals need to make a decision on each occasion about whether it's acceptable to lie or not. One factor highlighted in the earlier discussion was the question of who benefits from the deception, since there's a big difference between lying to someone as a kindness to them and lying for one's own convenience. There are many situations where both parties will benefit from a deception. For instance, saying that medication for a complex and potentially worrying medical condition is *just to help you sleep* could ensure it is accepted, which helps both the person and the carer. But when it's a competition, who should win? It is the unimpaired person who gets to choose.

We can see that benefiting from a deception at the expense of the person living with the dementia is questionable. But we also need to keep in mind how deceiving a person living with a dementia for their benefit can be costly for the other person. Lying, even when it will have a positive effect, can instil guilt. Wondering whether to tell the truth or not can become an agony. A lot is being asked of families and carers when they have to navigate the path between truth and deception. Many end up realizing that 'truth-dumping' (telling the truth on principle, even if the person won't be able to cope with it) is an indulgence they must forgo. Deception is often an act of love and self-denial, as a family member or carer accepts their own discomfort as a price to be paid for supporting the emotional wellbeing of the person living with the dementia.

ACTION POINTS FOR PEOPLE LIVING WITH A DEMENTIA

1. Think about times when you've said something untrue to someone. Why did you do it? Did you feel guilty? Imagine some change to the details of that situation that means you'd have felt differently.
2. Look back at the six scenarios on page 158. For each one, how would you feel about being lied to if you were that person living with the dementia?
3. Could you have a conversation with someone you trust about your views on being deceived now, and in the future? You could tell them that you understand the challenges they might face in the future. And you could outline what sort of approach you'd prefer.

ACTION POINTS FOR FAMILIES, FRIENDS AND PROFESSIONALS

1. Think about times when you've said something untrue to a person living with a dementia or haven't corrected something untrue that they believed. Why did you do it and how did you feel? Are there any patterns in what you consider acceptable versus unacceptable deception?
2. Choose two of the scenarios on page 158 and work out as many different approaches as possible for how they could be handled, both using deception and not using it. For each approach think about what might happen next, and how you and the person living with the dementia might feel.
3. Discuss the issue of deception with other people in your situation. To what extent do you agree with each other?

4. What's your best guess about whether the person living with a dementia you care for would accept being deceived if it were for good reason? Can you think of any way of finding out more from them?

ACTION POINTS FOR BYSTANDERS

1. Do you think it's easier or harder for someone in your position to be untruthful to a person living with a dementia than it is for someone who's with them more consistently and frequently? Why?
2. Thinking of the different people living with a dementia whom you've encountered, would you treat them all the same way if faced with the same question about whether to be truthful or not? If not, what is it about each person that would influence your decision about what to do?
3. If a family member or close professional carer asked you to collaborate with them in sustaining the deception of a person living with a dementia, what considerations would shape whether you did or not?

CHAPTER NINE

Making Communication Work Better

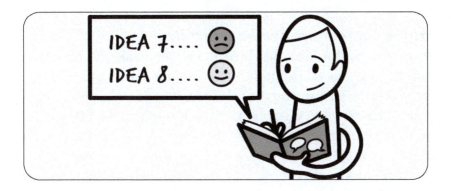

Empowering our conversations

At the end of a six-week *Empowered Conversations* workshop on communicating with people living with a dementia, participants commented on how the workshops had altered their understanding of dementia communication for the better. Belinda expressed surprise about the core problem that dementia causes: 'I always thought of it as memory...but no, it was communication and I was struck by that, because that immediately enables [me] to cope, because... it is something that I do.' Jenny, talking about her father living with a dementia said: 'He's not in a position to have control, but I did try to...give him a bit more choice in things, rather than just saying you're doing this.' Kate, reflecting on why her father struggled to join in large gatherings, commented: 'We realized now, he needed to be sat with the people he knew and to be close to them [rather] than be further down the table with family that he doesn't generally talk to.'[1]

In similar vein, this final chapter asks what can be done, at a practical level, to improve communication when one of the participants is living with a dementia. As the quotes above suggest, it's often small changes that can make a big difference. Belinda points out that since dementia is, in so many respects, a *communication disease*,[2] we have lots of scope for altering the status quo, because communication is something we do jointly. We may not be able to improve someone's memory, but simply by changing what *we* do in communication we can create opportunities for the other person to respond differently.

Why is communication so difficult?

It's easy to get the idea that dementia is what makes communication difficult. But that's not the whole story by any means. Blaming the disease is like blaming the pebble on the road when you fall off your unicycle while juggling six balls and balancing a flowerpot on your head. Yes, it's the pebble that toppled you off, but the real culprit is the difficulty of what you were trying to do at the time.

Communication is *always* hard, right through our lives. It's just that we have years of experience and lots of flexibility to help us cope with the most common issues when they arise. Sometimes, we barely notice there's been a problem at all. For instance, if we don't quite follow what someone said, we just ask them to repeat it. We might misunderstand what someone intended and be momentarily confused, before laughing and saying, *Oh, I thought you meant...!*

Meanwhile, it's not just in the dementia context that major breakdowns in communication can occur. Even without dementia in the picture, friends can vow never to speak to each other again because of some perceived, but unintended, slight. Planes crash because the

---

1   These comments were made in feedback interviews conducted after Empowered Conversations workshops in 2019 and early 2020 and are reproduced with the permission of the participants (names have been changed). Empowered Conversations was developed in Salford, UK, by Six Degrees Social Enterprise and is affiliated with Age Concern (https:// empowered-conversations.co.uk).

2   Wray (2018)

pilot misinterpreted the controller's instructions. Politicians express a view clumsily in a tweet and lose their job.

The reason communication so often goes wrong is that we have to balance many bits of information and we don't always get it right. We've seen in this book that all of the following have to be handled in real time: sounds (or movements in sign language, or letter shapes in writing), words, phrases and expressions, sentences, explicit meanings, implicit meanings, contexts and intentions. Speakers have to decide what they want to achieve. They also have to work out what to say in order to maximize the chances of achieving it. That means assessing what listeners are able to see, hear and understand, what they're likely to expect and think reasonable, and how they might respond to the different possible ways of presenting the message. For example, is shouting going to make them *more* likely to respond in the desired way, or *less* likely to? There are no hard-and-fast rules for these judgements. They depend on how well the speaker can assess the specific situation on that occasion with that person.

Listeners have a lot of work to do as well. They have to pay attention if they're to identify the words and make sense of them. Then they have to work out why the words were said in that way and thus what the speaker intended. That involves some mental acrobatics. The listener needs to guess what the speaker guessed about *their* knowledge and beliefs. For example, suppose the speaker says, ... *and it was* FIVE-*nil in the end.* Built into that statement are lots of assumptions that the listener has to recognize and process, such as: you're talking about a soccer game; it's a particular game that you believe I'm likely to think of first; five goals is a quantity you believe I don't already know about and am not expecting, and so on.

Once we recognize how very complicated ordinary communication is, it's a lot easier to see why dementia can cause additional problems. In particular, dementia makes it more difficult for people to take in, recall and/or assemble information in the way they used to. As a result, often neither they nor the person they're interacting with will have full confidence that messages are going to pass successfully between them. They're right not to have full confidence. Missing information means that each person has different beliefs and assumptions about what's relevant and what's known by the other person – and that increases the chances of people talking at cross-purposes. Losing confidence can then have onward effects. People enter more tentatively into conversations, worried about what might go wrong. Or they sit on a knife-edge of frustration and anger about not being able to communicate better – something that the other person could easily misinterpret as negativity towards them personally.

What can we do to make communication work better?

There are lots of things that can be done to improve the chances of successful communication when one of the participants is living with a dementia. And although much of the responsibility must fall on those whose abilities are not impaired, there are some steps that people living with a dementia can take for themselves. Indeed, it's important for *everyone* to feel they can play their part in helping themselves and the other person. So, here are some pointers for practical changes we can make.

Be curious about how communication works and why it can go wrong

It's easy to get into a position where we feel that we're failing or that the other person is. In that situation, frustration and disappointment come to the surface and can colour and shape what happens next. Instead, we can take an interest in what might have gone wrong. Doing so will help us stay relatively light-hearted about the situation so we can be more constructive in our approach. By becoming 'detectives', we place ourselves in a position of strength and power to make effective changes. Here are two checklists to help pin down what might have gone wrong if communication isn't working. The first concerns what can go wrong when the unimpaired person is the speaker and the person living with the dementia is the listener. The second checklist is for the reverse arrangement.

CHECKLIST 1 – FOR THE UNIMPAIRED PERSON AS SPEAKER

What you said:

- How clearly did you express yourself?
- Did you um and er a lot?
- Did you change direction part-way through, making it hard to follow the message?
- Did you speak quietly or very quickly?
- Were you facing away?
- Was there background noise competing with your speech?
- Did you get the attention of the person living with the dementia before you started?

How you said it:

- Did your tone of voice, body language or facial expression convey frustration, or anger? Sometimes, how you say something will be the main message a person living with a dementia picks up, carrying more weight than the words.

Context:

- Did you start a new topic without warning, so the person wasn't yet tuned into the context?
- Did you make assumptions about what they might know or remember that perhaps weren't accurate?
- Were they tuning into a different time or place from you (such as something in the past)?

Expectations:

- How did you expect the person living with the dementia to respond to what you said?
- Does what happened instead give you hints about what they thought you intended?
- Were your expectations reasonable and practical? For example, have you accepted that they may not be able to respond as they used to? If so, notice how that makes you feel.

Help the person living with the dementia to help themselves:

- If applicable, ensure they're wearing their hearing aids and glasses.
- Allow them time to process what you're saying.
- Notice indications that they don't understand and make changes as soon as you can.
- Be alert to their not having tuned in at the start – you may simply need to begin again now you have their attention.
- If they ask for clarification, provide it willingly and without frustration. This will encourage them to continue investing in the conversation. Otherwise, they may give up and switch off, or else become stressed and anxious or feel rejected.

CHECKLIST 2 – FOR THE UNIMPAIRED PERSON AS LISTENER

Assumptions:

- When the person living with the dementia started to speak, what did you assume they were going to say and mean? Might your assumptions have been wrong?

Evaluation:

- What might the person hope to achieve by speaking to you? Are you able to provide what they want? (Remember, the real reason might not be the most obvious one. For example, asking what time it is might indicate anxiety, so that they need reassurance more than information.)

What they said:

- If their statement doesn't make sense or is incorrect, can you work out what beliefs and assumptions they were working from?

How they said it:

- If the words or phrases they use don't make sense, might

they have substituted one word for another? Can you help them explain what they meant? One strategy is to reflect back what they just said, to see how they then expand on it. For example: 'Mum once said to me that she had two sons and no daughters. I reflected back her statement like I had no idea about her sons (which in this case I didn't!): "Oh, so you only have two sons and no daughters?" That led her to talk about her two brothers, which is what she really intended to say'.[3]

Help the person living with the dementia to help themselves:

- Be sensitive to how they feel about struggling to express messages effectively and make changes to their world.
- Encourage them to have another go, by being patient and by engaging in 'indirect repair' (described on page 171).
- Notice how you feel if you can't help them change their world as they hoped.

Develop empathy

We saw in Chapter 7 that we are more likely to treat people living with dementia kindly if we have empathy with them. That means we need to recognize, one way or another, something of what they are going through. There are various virtual-reality and immersive experiences that simulate the confusing sounds, images and information that people living with a dementia have to deal with. One powerful example I've seen is getting someone to make a cup of tea in a darkened kitchen that they're not familiar with (so they don't know which cupboards to look in, or even if all the things they need will be there), while wearing goggles that obscure their vision, headphones that blank out relevant sounds and create distracting noises, heavy boots, and thick rubber gloves that make it hard to manipulate objects. It's less about whether these various impediments directly reflect what a particular person living with a dementia is experiencing, than about

---

3   Maria Nicol, personal communication

how quickly someone hampered in this way experiences a sense of powerlessness, anxiety and panic.

It's these strong emotions that we need to recognize as central to the dementia experience – emotions arising from lacking control of even basic things, not being understood, losing the capacity to hang on to the information needed for making sense of situations and being rejected or sidelined by others. The reason we need to think about what it's like to be in that situation is because this is how we develop the most appropriate type of empathy – *response-based empathy* (Chapter 7).

This is the type of empathy that locks us into how another person is reacting to a situation, rather than what the situation is. They may have hooked their anxiety onto something that wouldn't make us anxious at all. But so what? If they're anxious, they're anxious. If they're still anxious even after we've reassured them about whatever they *said* they're anxious about, then their anxiety may well come from a deeper place and require a different kind of reassurance. The more we can spot emotional responses that we recognize, even if in us they would be caused by something else, the more we'll be able to tune into how people living with a dementia are feeling and meet them where they are.

Imagine what the person living with the dementia may be thinking

People living with a dementia are first and foremost people. They may well have lived a long life in which they were a successful communicator, an effective worker, a valued family member and a dear friend. Perhaps they chaired committees, dealt with difficult customers, explained complicated issues. Now, their communication is going wrong. They are likely to feel inept and foolish about making mistakes, being misunderstood, and being less and less able to do things for themselves.[4] They may think that others despise them

---

4   For a valuable insight into these experiences, see the chapter called 'Alzheimer's Disease: The Subjective Experience' in *Alzheimer's Disease and Dementia: What Everyone Needs to Know* (Sabat 2018).

for it or are annoyed with them. They may think others find them a nuisance and would prefer not to deal with them.

With less information being stored, they will sometimes be confused about what they're supposed to know. They might feel as if knowledge is seeping through their fingers like sand. They might feel they can't keep up. If so, even if they desperately want to be part of things, they may be tempted to sit quietly and not try to engage, in case they get something wrong or can't cope. They could be in a swirl of distressing emotions. People living with a dementia might spend a lot of time thinking about the predicament they're in, feeling unable to do much about it, and not knowing how to ask for help, or what help to ask for.

One thing we can do is listen and watch more attentively. Like anyone else, people living with a dementia may not always say very directly what they're thinking and feeling – they may not even fully understand it all. Add to that their difficulties with using language and holding information together and it may take some detective work to see what they want to convey.

Steven Sabat uses a technique called 'indirect repair'[5] to help pin down someone's meaning. This approach involves attending carefully to what's said, making a reasonable guess in the light of the context, and then saying it back to the person, to check if it's what they intended. This way, it's possible to support people living with a dementia towards expressing ideas that they can't quite produce. Importantly, it signals to them that you're trying as hard as you can to help them say what they want to. Here's an example of how Sabat achieves this in practice, in conversation with one of his clients, Dr B:[6]

> *Dr B: Uh [5 second pause] I, I take a lot of [3.1 sec.] things [2.9 sec.] that I feel are [5.6 sec.], uh, there fear, there are, been, things that I would, should do, you now, but it doesn't, it hasn't ever, you know, come through. I don't know, I don't know what I'm talking about*

---

5   See Sabat (2018, p. 96ff).
6   Sabat (2001, pp. 30–31)

Sabat: Oh yes – I think you do. I think I know. May I try to tell you what I think you're talking about?

Dr B: *What*

Sabat: You're saying that you feel there are things you should be able to do

Dr B: *Yeah*

Sabat: And you don't seem to be able to do them

Dr B: *Yeah*

Sabat: What sorts of things?

In this example, Sabat is proactive in suggesting what Dr B meant. However, it's not an attempt to take over so Dr B is silenced. Rather, it's a gateway for Dr B. There are several things that Sabat does to make that that happen. First, he asks permission before he makes his guess. Second, he keeps his suggestions simple, and waits to check that Dr B agrees with what he's said (this of course involves also checking facial expression and body language). And then Sabat uses the shared knowledge as the springboard to get additional information. In this way, he propels Dr B into a new opportunity to talk about his problems and how he's experiencing them. This wouldn't have been possible if Sabat had simply nodded and said *uhuh*, however sympathetically that was done.

Consider what people living with a dementia might most urgently want to change in their world

I've suggested in this book that when we communicate with others, it's because we want to make some sort of change to our world that we can't make without their help. If we fail to achieve that change, we'll feel powerless and frustrated. Many of us will have experienced this from time to time. I recall once trying to buy cubed stewing steak in a shop in Germany. I didn't know the name for that cut of meat, so I just pointed at what I wanted in the array of meat products on display. Unfortunately, the assistant thought I'd pointed to something else and started weighing out minced (ground) beef instead. I'd have liked to explain and get her to change what she was weighing, but I didn't feel confident enough about my German to risk doing so. Instead, I just gave in and accepted what she sold me. Luckily, it was still something I could use even though I had to find a different recipe. But I felt stupid and defeated.

How unpleasant it must be if, day after day, and in relation to many things that matter a great deal more than how finely cut up your meat is, a person feels defeated like that. For them it may mean they can't get pain relief, or information, or reassurance. We might be able to help them, if we're observant enough to notice that something has gone wrong, take a guess about what, and use that to help them explain what they need.

It's not easy to get inside someone's head and work out what they meant to achieve when they communicated, and we won't always get it right. But two things can give us clues. One is what the person actually did say (or do), even if it's not quite what they needed to say or do to achieve their purpose. The other is the context in which it was said, and our understanding of what other contexts the person might be taking into account. Here's an example.

Suppose a person living with a dementia asks you how your dog is, but you don't have a dog. In deciding how to reply, there are various things to consider. Is it possible the wrong word came out, and they meant to ask about your cat, horse or son, say? Context may help you decide. For instance, do they (like Val's dad in Chapter 5) often muddle up words like this? Has anything just occurred that might have put the idea, or the false word, in their mind? Alternatively, could they have mistaken you for someone else? We need to be wary of taking offence. We've all mistaken one person for another at some point, and it's awkward and embarrassing for both parties. Handling it lightly will help.

The key to how to respond is to figure out what the person was trying to achieve by asking the question. Was it an expression of interest? Of concern? Or was it just a way to start a conversation? In any of these cases, replying, *What are you talking about? I don't have a dog!* won't help them achieve their goal. If they seem to want specific information, you might reply, *Well, I don't have a dog, but I wonder if you meant my cat? She's a lot better now, thanks.* Even if you've guessed wrongly, you've given value to the enquiry, so the focus isn't on the miscommunication. And if you think they're just being sociable, you might say, *Well, I don't have a dog, but if I did, I'd have a poodle. What would you have?* This gets a conversation going, and it's a more positive and constructive response than just telling them they're wrong. It makes light of the mismatch in belief and moves the focus onto something that's easier to manage. If the person living with the dementia realizes they made a mistake about your having a dog, they might feel embarrassed, but they'll be heartened that it doesn't seem to bother you and that the conversation has shifted away from that mistake.

There are also more systematic things we can do to improve our understanding of how people living with a dementia would like to improve their world. One is *asking them*! In *Dancing with Dementia*,[7] Christine Bryden describes co-organizing a workshop in which people who, like her, were living with a dementia were put into one discussion group and their family members into another. Both groups considered the same topics. One topic was how well the family member(s) understood what the person living with the dementia was feeling. After the discussion, the groups came back and reported to each other. This exercise seems to have been quite an eye-opener for both groups. Family members discovered that the people living with a dementia generally thought 'the family didn't really understand what it was like not to remember the most ordinary and everyday things'. Families didn't always realize what was most important to the people living with a dementia: 'What we all wanted was to be listened to, to be asked what our wishes were.' One participant explained how his wife now did everything for him, which made him feel useless. Importantly, he didn't want to say anything in case he upset her.[8] That's something to keep in mind – people living with a dementia will often be very sensitive to the burden they are placing on others, and not want to appear ungrateful by mentioning issues that arise.

---

7   Bryden (2005)
8   Bryden (2005, pp. 44–45)

Build social and emotional reserve

As described in Chapter 2, a person's experience when living with a dementia, or caring for someone who does, can be considerably improved if they have high social and emotional reserve. Social reserve is the support someone has from society, including timely and helpful information, joined-up services, social interaction and positive attitudes. A person enjoying high social reserve will be more likely to also build high emotional reserve – that is, they will be more able to cope with challenges without falling into anxiety or depression.

We can all do our bit to increase people's social and emotional reserve, by offering practical and moral support. We can also demand that politicians provide effective health and social infrastructure and prioritize the welfare of people living with a dementia, their families and care professionals.

Think about the pros and cons of lying

In Chapter 8, I suggested that there isn't a simple answer to the question *Is it okay to deceive a person living with a dementia?* The reason is that each situation is different, with its own considerations to be balanced out, including whether hearing the truth would upset the person; how they'd feel if they found out about the deception; whether the main beneficiary of the lie is you or them; and what the possible longer-term consequences are of lying versus not lying.

The consensus in recent writing on the topic of lying to people living with a dementia is that it's not something to do lightly or to use to take advantage of them. A good rule of thumb is to first consider being truthful. Occasionally, the truth will be upsetting for the person, but that doesn't always mean it should be avoided – sadness is a legitimate feeling to have sometimes. However, if after proper reflection we consider deception to be the kindest way forward on a particular occasion, because it'll protect the person from physical danger or from deep emotions they can't handle, then that option shouldn't be ruled out purely because we're squeamish about lying. Although we must be careful about comparing people living with a dementia with children, in this particular regard, the way we approach lying to children might be a helpful guide. There won't ever be a single rule, and each situation needs evaluating in its own right.

The main thing to be aware of is that deception is a complex and troubling matter, and so if you feel guilty about telling a lie, or indeed about not doing so, it shouldn't surprise you, and you shouldn't feel that you are in some way managing the situation less well than others would.

Holding on to a sense of identity

In Chapters 4 and 7 we saw that dementia can easily eat away at a person's sense of identity. People living with a dementia might struggle to recall events in their own life that others can recall, which means they have less ownership than others do of things that happened to them. Fear of forgetting who we are might be one of the most fundamental fears humans can have. We need to support people living with a dementia in anchoring aspects of their identity, by encouraging them to reminisce, reminding them of people, events and skills they once knew about, and reassuring them that they still 'own' this information.

Family carers can also feel they're losing their identity, particularly if their caring responsibilities prevent them from undertaking activities they used to enjoy, seeing friends and visiting favourite places. It's important for family carers to find ways of continuing to have a life beyond that role. This is an element of social reserve that all of us can help to build for each other. Picking up the phone to chat to a friend or neighbour who's caring for someone living with a dementia could help them find a part of themselves that isn't 'carer'. And helping them go out on their own to do things for themselves will be hugely beneficial. It might involve offering to sit with the person living with the dementia for a while or giving them both a lift to a place where they can separately follow their own interests. Financial support for charities that create such opportunities is another way to help.

Next, we'll consider another element of identity. It's one that all of us can reflect on, particularly in relation to the challenges of communication.

Who shall I be today?

In different situations, we often take on slightly different personal characteristics. For instance, we might be very chatty and outgoing when we're in one group of people, yet be quiet in another group. We might be willing to take the lead and organize things in one setting, but be reluctant to put ourselves forward in another. The reasons can be complex, often reflecting how others are behaving towards us. But it shows we can be more than one thing – we can act in more than one way.

Years ago, I used to visit an elderly lady whose life wasn't easy, because of disability and bereavement. Yet she was always cheerful, friendly and interested in others. One day, I asked how she managed to be so positive, given what she was going through. She replied, 'I've learnt over the years that it's wise to be cheerful and kind. You feel better. And other people want to spend time with you. So you're less miserable and less alone.'

What she taught me was that being cheerful and kind is a choice. Before, I'd assumed we could only react to how we felt. But she was *choosing* to behave as if she were cheerful, and the positive feelings followed. I'm sure she still felt despondent at times. But she had a strategy that gave her some control. Being cheerful with other people meant they wanted her company, which then supported her. By reaching out to others, she built up their emotional and social reserve and also her own.

Life is very challenging for people living with a dementia and those supporting them. There may be times when it seems that there's no alternative to enduring negative experiences like weariness, frustration, sadness, disappointment and anger. It might seem impossible to reconnect with lasting feelings of joy or hope. But realizing that we're flexible in how we respond in situations is the key to finding ways out of patterns of communication that aren't working.

If we feel frustrated every time we communicate with a particular person, that's because we've got stuck in the *I'm a frustrated person* mode. It will, of course, seem at the time as if it's unavoidable, because they're always so frustrating! How else could we respond? But try this test. Think of three people you know – say, a good friend, a younger relative and an acquaintance. Now imagine each of them saying or doing whatever it was that made you frustrated. You're likely to find that you wouldn't feel equally frustrated with each of them, even though they said or did the same thing. Nor would you, probably, respond in the same way. That's because we have more than one option for how we respond to something.

The choices we make about how to respond reflect how we understand the context (see Chapters 4 and 5). An important part of that context is the assumptions and beliefs we have about the other person and about ourselves. If we can just question these, we're in a position to adjust them – and this is something we can all try, whether we're living with a dementia or supporting someone who is. For instance, if we've fixed in our mind that a particular person doesn't care about us, we might only tend to choose negative, defensive options. If we start to notice and re-evaluate the assumptions, we may realize that those assumptions aren't reliable or accurate any more (if they ever were). That could open up a new set of possible ways to respond.

Experimenting with different approaches is worth a try. It might well generate positive feelings. And it will change the context for the other person, giving them more options for how to respond. Armed with an awareness that we're capable of responding in more than one way in a situation, we can begin to ask ourselves, *Who am I being today?* and *Is this who I want to be today?* For instance, instead of being someone who's too busy to sit down for a minute, we could be someone who feels that sitting with another person is time well spent. Instead of being someone who's anxious, we could be someone who looks for the funny side of situations. Instead of being someone who's gloomy about things, we could be someone who's positive and cheerful.

This doesn't mean that interacting with people living with a dementia requires us to be constantly chirpy and to deny the feelings we have. It simply means that it's helpful if we can notice how we're reacting. If we have negative feelings, that's part of what we need to notice. Our own responses to challenging situations, particularly in relation to communication breakdown, become another opportunity for us to be curious about what's happening. And this immediately gives us new ways to deal with how we feel.

Moving forward with kindness

Penelope Campling defines 'intelligent kindness' as 'not a soft, sentimental feeling or action' but 'a binding, creative and problem-solving force that inspires and focuses the imagination and goodwill'.[9] Acting with kindness isn't always easy, because our emotions can get in the way of seeing the full range of options for how to respond. That's why this book has aimed to offer insights into what happens when communication doesn't work. We need to give ourselves the chance to stand back and notice what's happening. Then we'll become curious about causes and effects, and we're less likely to feel anxious, frustrated or guilty when things don't go quite right.

The reason why breakdowns in communication so often result in strong emotions is that our aim in communicating is to make changes to our world that we can't make without someone else's help. Not achieving the outcomes we want is more than disappointing. It can feel frightening. If that's how it feels to us, then that's how it feels to people living with a dementia as well – and they may well experience these difficulties much more often.

Understanding the situation enables our empathy, and that will help us locate and draw on our deep well of intelligent kindness – towards others and ourselves. When we find that resource, we can use it to build up our own emotional reserve (Chapter 2) and everyone else's too. The stronger we all are emotionally, the greater our ability to offer the practical and moral support (social reserve, Chapter 2) that will help people deal with the inevitable challenges of their lives, whether they're living with a dementia or not.

---

9   Campling (2015, p. 4)

Social and emotional reserve need to be built and sustained not only for people living with a dementia but also those who support them daily. It's easy to overlook how complicated and challenging individual circumstances can be. The spouse of a person living with a dementia might well have their own health problems to deal with and could feel very alone if their lifelong partner is no longer able to support *them*. The children of people living with a dementia might be trying to help despite living a long way away and having a demanding job and/or their own family to care for. Other considerations include family relationships that are not always perfect, which can make it hard to ask relatives for help, while practical challenges are often made worse if there's not much money to spare. In addition, in minority ethnic communities, there can be taboos about dementia that make it hard to talk about. And there could be communication challenges due to limited language knowledge, on top of those associated with the dementia.[10]

If we're to support people living with a dementia and those who care for them into getting the best quality of life they can possibly have, we need to maximize their chances of being able to make the changes to their world that they want. That means giving them the opportunity to express their needs through effective, supportive communication. Since dementias undermine communication in various ways, we can't expect things to be straightforward all the time, but there are plenty of techniques – many mentioned in this book – for improving the chances that a person will successfully get their message across. Our focus, as we approach them with respect and kindness, needs to be wondering what they would like to change – or protect from changing – in their world. To do that, we need to sufficiently glimpse how their world looks, and find a way to align it with our own.

---

10   Wray (2020a) is an animated film about ways of addressing these challenges.

ACTION POINTS FOR PEOPLE LIVING WITH A DEMENTIA

1. Do you think that others understand how you feel and what you need? Could you discuss with them your concerns about being misunderstood? Perhaps you have some ideas for how things could be improved. If you don't want to talk to them directly, could you write your thoughts down and show them?

2. Could you develop curiosity about your own predicaments in living with your dementia? If you take an interest in what happens and why, it might help you come up with different choices about what occurs next.

3. To what extent do you get frustrated with another person, when in fact you're frustrated with dementia? Experiment with being cheerful and appreciative, and see if that changes how they respond.

ACTION POINTS FOR FAMILIES, FRIENDS AND PROFESSIONALS

1. Next time you're in a situation where the communication hasn't worked as you expected, try stepping back and asking what really happened? This may help you avoid giving an immediate emotional response. You may notice ways to improve the situation in future. For instance, you might realize you used an unhelpful tone, spoke too fast or didn't pay attention to what the person was trying to achieve when they spoke.

2. Rerun in your mind some situations that have occurred, trying out different ways you could have responded (e.g. smiling, giving the person a hug, walking out of the room for a while, laughing, changing the subject). How easy is it for you to guess how the other person would have responded if you'd done each one? The aim is to experiment with breaking old patterns (such as sounding annoyed, negative body language, automatically contradicting them). If you can identify one or two alternative

responses that seem possible in your situation, why not try them out in a future conversation and see what happens?

3. If you're a family carer and you know someone in a similar situation to your own, why not bring the two households together for a day? Experiment with supporting the other person's loved one, to see how similar and different it feels. Notice whether you have different emotional reactions when interacting with a person you haven't got close emotional bonds with.

ACTION POINTS FOR BYSTANDERS

1. A risk for those who don't spend much time with people living with a dementia is that they develop just one approach, which they always use with that person and perhaps with every such person they meet. It might work okay (e.g. having a light chat about the weather and how they are), but it's still a set pattern, and perhaps you've already found it quite limiting. Why not experiment with some alternatives? To get ideas, observe what other people do.

2. If you meet the same person living with a dementia regularly, see if you can draw out a different aspect of them each time you meet them. For example, can you get them to laugh? Can you find out something new about their life? Can you find out what their favourite colour is? Each new opportunity they have to connect with you could help build up their social and emotional reserve.

References

Abraha, I., Rimland, J.M., Lozano-Montoya, I., Dell'Aquila, G. et al. (2020). Simulated presence therapy of dementia. *Cochrane Database of Systematic Reviews 4*, CD011882. doi:10.1002/14651858.CD011882.pub3.

Alladi, S., Bak, T.H., Duggirala, V., Surampudi, B. et al. (2013). Bilingualism delays age at onset of dementia, independent of education and immigration status. *Neurology 81*, 1938-1944.

Alzheimer's Society (2020). Alzheimer's Society's view on specialised early care for Alzheimer's. Retrieved from www.alzheimers.org.uk/about-us/policy-and-influencing/what-we-think/specialised-early-care-alzheimers-specal

Bailey, S., Scales, K., Lloyd, J., Schneider, J. and Jones, R. (2015). The emotional labour of health-care assistants in inpatient dementia care. *Ageing and Society 35*, 2, 246-269.

Balbag, M.A., Pedersen, N.L. and Gatz, M. (2014). Playing a musical instrument as a protective factor against dementia and cognitive impairment: A population-based twin study. *International Journal of Alzheimer's Disease 2014*, 836748. doi:10.1155/2014/836748

Bartrés-Faz, D. and Arenaza-Urquijo, E.M. (2011). Structural and functional imaging correlates of cognitive and brain reserve hypotheses in healthy and pathological aging. *Brain Topography 24*, 3-4, 340-357.

Baum, S. and Titone, D. (2014). Moving toward a neuroplasticity view of bilingualism, executive control, and aging. *Applied Psycholinguistics 35*, 5, 857-894.

Bialystok, E., Craik, F.I.M. and Freedman, M. (2007). Bilingualism as a protection against the onset of symptoms of dementia. *Neuropsychologia 45*, 2, 459-464.

Bowlby, M.C. (1991). Reality orientation thirty years later: Are we still confused? *Canadian Journal of Occupational Therapy 58*, 3, 114-122.

Brown, M. and Clegg, D. (Eds) (2007). *Ancient Mysteries*. London: Trebus Project. www.trebusprojects.org

Bryden, C. (2005). *Dancing with Dementia*. London: Jessica Kingsley Publishers.

Bute, J. (2010). *Understanding My Dementia*. Retrieved from http://gloriousopportunity.org/resources/Understanding_My_Dementia.pdf

Caiazza, R., James, I.A., Rippon, D., Grossi, D. and Cantone, D. (2016). Should we tell lies to people with dementia in their best interest? The views of Italian and English medical doctors. *Faculty of the Psychology of Older People Bulletin 134*, April, 35-40.

Camberg, L., Woods, P., Ooi, W.L., Hurley, A., et al. (1999). Evaluation of Simulated Presence: A personalized approach to enhance well-being in persons with Alzheimer's disease. *Journal of the American Geriatrics Society 47*, 4, 446-452.

Campling, P. (2015). Reforming the culture of healthcare: The case for intelligent kindness. *BJPsych Bulletin 39*, 1, 1-5.

Chertkow, H., Whitehead, V., Phillips, N., Wolfson, C., Atherton, J. and Bergman, H. (2010). Multilingualism (but not always bilingualism) delays the onset of Alzheimer disease: Evidence from a bilingual community. *Alzheimer Disease & Associated Disorders 24*, 2, 118-125.

Clare, L., Whitaker, C.J., Craik, F.I.M., Bialystok, E. et al. (2016). Bilingualism, executive control, and age at diagnosis among people with early-stage Alzheimer's disease in Wales. *Journal of Neuropsychology 10*, 163–185.

Clegg, D. (2010). *Tell Mrs Mill Her Husband Is Still Dead*. London: Trebus Project. www.trebusprojects.org

Clegg, D. (2015). *An Occasional Cobra*. London: Trebus Project. Retrieved from www.trebusprojects.org/an-occasional-cobra

Comas-Herrera, A. and Knapp, M. (2016). *Cognitive Stimulation Therapy (CST): Summary of Evidence on Cost-effectiveness*. Retrieved from www.england.nhs.uk/wp-content/uploads/2018/01/dg-cognitive-stimulation-therapy.pdf

Davis, B.H. and Maclagan, M. (2010). Formulaicity, Pauses and Fillers in Alzheimer's Discourse: Gluing Relationships as Impairment Increases. In N. Amiridze, B. Davis and M. Maclagan (Eds), *Fillers, Pauses and Placeholders* (pp. 189–216). Amsterdam: John Benjamins.

Davis, B.H. and Maclagan, M. (2013). 'Aw, so how's your day going?': Ways That Persons with Dementia Keep their Conversational Partner Involved. In B. Davis and J. Guendouzi (Eds), *Pragmatics in Dementia Discourse* (pp. 83–116). Newcastle-upon-Tyne: Cambridge Scholars Publishing.

Day, A.M., James, I.A., Meyer, T.D. and Lee, D.R. (2011). Do people with dementia find lies and deception in dementia care acceptable? *Aging & Mental Health 15*, 7, 822–829.

de Bot, K. (2017). The Future of the Bilingual Advantage. In S.E. Pfenniger and J. Navracsics (Eds), *Future Research Directions for Applied Linguistics* (pp. 15–32). Bristol: Multilingual Matters.

Dementia Care Matters (2016). The Butterfly Household model of care action checklist (revised version 2). Hove: Dementia Care Matters.

Deters, K.D., Nho, K., Risacher, S.L., Kim, S. ... the Alzheimer's Disease Neuroimaging Initiative. (2017). Genome-wide association study of language performance in Alzheimer's disease. *Brain and Language 172*, 22–29.

Feil, N. (2009). Gladys Wilson and Naomi Feil. www.youtube.com/watch?v=CrZXz10FcVM

Gallagher, P. (2018, 23 March). 'What they saw reduced care staff to tears': This Dutch dementia village could arrive in Kent by 2020. *i-news*. Retrieved from https://inews.co.uk/news/health/dutch-dementia-village-kent-england

Gaser, C. and Schlaug, G. (2003). Brain structures differ between musicians and non-musicians. *Journal of Neuroscience 23*, 27, 9240–9245.

Godel, M. (2000). A SPECAL way of maintaining well-being in dementia. *Journal of Dementia Care 8*, 5, 20–23.

Gollan, T.H., Salmon, D.P., Montoya, R.I. and Galasko, D.R. (2011). Degree of bilingualism predicts age of diagnosis of Alzheimer's disease in low-education but not in highly educated Hispanics. *Neuropsychologia 49*, 3826–3830.

Graves, A.B., Mortimer, J.A., Larson, E.B., Wenzlow, A., Bowen, J.D. and McCormick, W.C. (1996). Head circumference as a measure of cognitive reserve: Association with severity of impairment in Alzheimer's disease. *British Journal of Psychiatry 169*, 1, 86–92.

Guendouzi, J. (2013). So What's Your Name? Relevance in Dementia. In B. Davis and J. Guendouzi (Eds), *Pragmatics in Dementia Discourse* (pp. 29–54). Newcastle-upon-Tyne: Cambridge Scholars Publishing.

Guendouzi, J. and Savage, M. (2017). Alzheimer's Disease. In L. Cummings (Ed.), *Research in Clinical Pragmatics* (pp. 323–346). New York: Springer.

Hamilton, H.E. (2008). Narrative as snapshot: Glimpses into the past in Alzheimer's discourse. *Narrative Inquiry 18*, 1, 53–82.

Hillis, A.E., Oh, S. and Ken, L. (2004). Deterioration of naming nouns versus verbs in primary progressive aphasia. *Annals of Neurology 55*, 2, 268–275.

Hodges, J.R., Patterson, K., Oxbury, S. and Funnell, E. (1992). Semantic dementia: Progressive fluent aphasia with temporal lobe atrophy. *Brain 115*, 1783–1806.

Hudziak, J.J., Albaugh, M.D., Ducharme, S., Karama, S. et al. (2014). Cortical thickness maturation and duration of music training: Health-promoting activities shape brain development. *Journal of the American Academy of Child and Adolescent Psychiatry 53*, 11, 1153–1161.

Hyde, K.L., Lerch, J., Norton, A., Forgeard, M. et al. (2009). The effects of musical training on structural brain development: A longitudinal study. *Annals of the New York Academy of Sciences 1169*, 182–186.

James, I., Wood-Mitchell, A.J., Waterworth, A.M., Mackenzie, L.E. and Cunningham, J. (2006). Lying to people with dementia: Developing ethical guidelines for care settings. *International Journal of Geriatric Psychiatry 21*, 800–801.

James, O. (2008). *Contented Dementia*. London: Vermilion.

Katzman, R., Terry, R., DeTeresa, R., Brown, T. et al. (1988). Clinical, pathological, and neurochemical changes in dementia: A subgroup with preserved mental status and numerous neocortical plaques. *Annals of Neurology 23*, 2, 138–144.

Kirtley, A. and Williamson, T. (2016). *What Is Truth? An Inquiry about Truth and Lying in Dementia Care*. London: Mental Health Foundation. Retrieved from www.mentalhealth.org.uk/publications/what-truth-inquiry-about-truth-and-lying-dementia-care

Kitwood, T. (1997). *Dementia Reconsidered*. Maidenhead: Open University Press.

Klosterman, C. (2014). Nursing-home pitfalls. *New York Times Magazine*, 2 March, p. 17. www.nytimes.com/2014/03/02/magazine/nursing-home-pitfalls.html

Lampedusa, G.T. (2007). *The Leopard* (A. Colquhoun, Trans.). London: Vintage. (Original work published 1958)

Lipinska, D. (2009). *Person-centred Counselling for People with Dementia*. London: Jessica Kingsley Publishers.

Livingston, G., Sommerlad, A., Orgeta, V., Costafreda, S.G. et al. (2017). *Dementia Prevention, Intervention, and Care*. London. The Lancet Commissions.

Locke, J. (1690). *An Essay Concerning Humane Understanding. Book 2: Of Ideas*. London: Thomas Basset. www.gutenberg.org/files/10615/10615-h/10615-h.htm

McElveen, T. (2015). Lying to people with dementia: Treacherous act or beneficial therapy? *Royal College of Psychiatrists Newsletter*, September.

McLean, A. (2007). *The Person in Dementia: A Study of Nursing Home Care in the US*. Toronto: Broadview Press.

Miesen, B.M.L. (1999). *Dementia in Close-up*. London: Routledge.

Moisse, K. (2012). Alzheimer's disease: Dutch village doubles as nursing home. ABC News. Retrieved from https://abcnews.go.com/Health/AlzheimersCommunity/alzheimers-disease-dutch-village-dubbed-truman-show-dementia/story?id=16103780

Morton, J.B. (2014). Sunny review casts a foreboding shadow over status quo bilingual advantage research. *Applied Psycholinguistics 35*, 5, 929–932.

Mukadam, N., Sommerlad, A. and Livingston, G. (2017). The relationship of bilingualism compared to monolingualism to the risk of cognitive decline or dementia: A systematic review and meta-analysis. *Journal of Alzheimer's Disease 58*, 45–54.

Namazi, K.H., Rosner, T.T. and Calkins, M.P. (1989). Visual barriers to prevent ambulatory Alzheimer's patients from exiting through an emergency door. *The Gerontologist 29*, 5, 699–702.

O'Connell, B., Gardner, A., Takase, M., Hawkins, M.T. et al. (2007). Clinical usefulness and feasibility of using reality orientation with patients who have dementia in acute care settings. *International Journal of Nursing Practice 13*, 182–192.

O'Sullivan, G. (2011). Ethical and effective: Approaches to residential care for people with dementia. *Dementia 12*, 1, 111–121.

Ormrod, V. (2019). *In My Father's Memory*. Blakeney: Holborn House.

Paap, K.R. and Greenberg, Z.I. (2013). There is no coherent evidence for a bilingual advantage in executive processing. *Cognitive Psychology 66*, 2, 232–258.

Perani, D., Farsad, M., Ballarini, T., Lubian, F., et al. (2017). The impact of bilingualism on brain reserve and metabolic connectivity in Alzheimer's dementia. *Proceedings of the National Academy of Sciences 114*, 7, 1690–1695.

Perneczky, R., Wagenpfeil, S., Lunetta, K.L., Cupples, L.A. et al. (2010). Head circumference, atrophy, and cognition. *Neurology 75*, 2, 137–142.

Planos, J. (2014). The Dutch village where everyone has dementia. *The Atlantic*, 14 November. www.theatlantic.com/health/archive/2014/11/the-dutch-village-where-everyone-has-dementia/382195

Posner, R. (1980). Semantics and Pragmatics of Sentence Connectives in Natural Language. In J.R. Searle, F. Kiefer and M. Bierwisch (Eds), *Speech Act Theory and Pragmatics* (pp. 168–203). Dortrecht: Reidel.

Pritchard, E.J. and Dewing, J. (1999). *An Evaluation of SPECAL: A Multi-method Evaluation of the SPECAL Service for People with Dementia*. Oxford: Royal College of Nursing Institute.

Ramanathan, V. (1997). *Alzheimer Discourse: Some Sociolinguistic Dimensions*. Mahwah, NJ: Lawrence Erlbaum Associates.

Reilly, J., Troche, J. and Grossman, M. (2011). Language Processing in Dementia. In A.E. Budson and N.W. Kowall (Eds), *Handbook of Alzheimer's Disease and Other Dementias* (pp. 336–368). Oxford: Blackwell.

Roberts, A. and Orange, J.B. (2013). Discourse in Lewy Body Spectrum Disorder. In B. Davis and J. Guendouzi (Eds), *Pragmatics in Dementia Discourse* (pp. 147–204). Newcastle-upon-Tyne: Cambridge Scholars Publishing.

Sabat, S.R. (2001). *The Experience of Alzheimer's Disease: Life Through a Tangled Veil*. Oxford: Blackwell.

Sabat, S.R. (2018). *Alzheimer's Disease and Dementia: What Everyone Needs to Know*. New York: Oxford University Press.

Sampson, T. (2014). Holland's dementia village revolutionises Alzheimer's caregiving. UTNE Reader. Retrieved from www.utne.com/community/holland-dementia-village-revolutionizes -alzheimer-caregiving

Smith, E., Lamb-Yorski, R., Thompson, A. and Grootveld, C. (2019). *This Is Our Story: A Qualitative Research Report on Living with Dementia*. Wellington: Litmus.

Staff, R.T., Hogan, M.J., Williams, D.S. and Whalley, L.J. (2018). Intellectual engagement and cognitive ability in later life (the 'use it or lose it' conjecture): Longitudinal, prospective study. *British Medical Journal 363*, k4925.

Stern, Y., Zarahn, E., Habeck, C., Holtzer, R. et al. (2008). A common neural network for cognitive reserve in verbal and object working memory in young but not old. *Cerebral Cortex 18*, 4, 959–967.

Swinton, J. (2012). *Dementia: Living in the Memories of God*. London: SCM Press.

Taylor, R. (2007). *Alzheimer's from the Inside Out*. Baltimore, MA: Health Professions Press.

Tulving, E. (2002). Episodic memory: From mind to brain. *Annual Review of Psychology 53*, 1–25.

Turner, A., Eccles, F., Keady, J., Simpson, J. and Elvish, R. (2016). The use of the truth and deception in dementia care amongst general hospital staff. *Aging & Mental Health 21*, 8, 862–869.

Valian, V. (2015). Bilingualism and cognition. *Bilingualism: Language and Cognition 18*, 1, 3–24.

Williamson, T. and Kirtley, A. (2016). *Dementia Truth Enquiry: Review of Evidence*. London: Mental Health Foundation. www.mentalhealth.org.uk/publications/what-truth-inquiry-about-truth-and-lying-dementia-care

Wray, A. (2002). *Formulaic Language and the Lexicon*. Cambridge: Cambridge University Press.

Wray, A. (2010). 'We've had a wonderful, wonderful thing': Formulaic interaction when an expert has dementia. *Dementia 9*, 4, 517–534.

Wray, A. (2017). *Understanding the Challenges of Dementia Communication*. Tony Robinson (narrator) and David Hallangen (illustrator). www.youtube.com/watch?v=u6cchefGn2M

Wray, A. (2018). *Dementia: The 'Communication Disease'*. Tony Robinson (narrator) and David Hallangen (illustrator). www.youtube.com/watch?v=6uu63PqWGaU

Wray, A. (2020a). *Dementia Communication Across Language Boundaries: Developing Language Awareness*. Tony Robinson (narrator) and David Hallangen (illustrator). www.youtube.com/watch?v=sblxPq3eQoc

Wray, A. (2020b). *The Dynamics of Dementia Communication*. New York: Oxford University Press.

Index

Footnotes are indicated with the letter 'n'. Names in *italics* refer to case studies.